Complete Dentures: The Legacy Prosthetic System

One book, one tree: In support of reforestation worldwide and to address the climate crisis, for every book sold Quintessence Publishing will plant a tree (https://onetreeplanted.org/).

Library of Congress Cataloging-in-Publication Data

Names: Rohrbach, Steffen, author.
Title: Complete dentures : the Legacy prosthetic system / Steffen Rohrbach.

Description: Batavia, IL : Quintessence Publishing Co, Inc, [2025] | Includes bibliographical references and index. | Summary: "Step-by-step guide to fabricating functional and esthetic complete dentures in daily practice"-- Provided by publisher.
Identifiers: LCCN 2025001148 | ISBN 9781647242183 (paperback)
Subjects: MESH: Denture, Complete | Dental Prosthesis--methods
Classification: LCC RK656 | NLM WU 530 | DDC 617.6/92--dc23/eng/20250320
LC record available at https://lccn.loc.gov/2025001148

QUINTESSENCE PUBLISHING
USA

Quintessence Publishing Co, Inc
411 N Raddant Road
Batavia, IL 60510
www.quintessence-publishing.com

5 4 3 2 1

Editor: Leah Huffman
Production: Angelina Schmelter
Design: Sue Zubek

Printed in the USA

COMPLETE DENTURES

The Legacy Prosthetic System

Steffen Rohrbach, ZT
Senior Director, Removable Prosthetics
Edmonds Dental Prosthetics
Springfield, Missouri

QUINTESSENCE PUBLISHING

Berlin | Chicago | Tokyo
Barcelona | London | Milan | Paris | Prague | Seoul | Warsaw
Beijing | Istanbul | Sao Paulo | Sydney | Zagreb

CONTENTS

FOREWORD

Over the years, respect for the treatment of the edentulous patient has been lost. While it may be true that partial or complete tooth loss is not to be expected until later stages of life, it does not change the fact that edentulism should be treated therapeutically when it occurs.

Edentulous patients are looking for professionals, they are looking for medical assistance, and they are looking for solutions to restore their quality of life. But the necessary knowledge and skills to treat them has increasingly been forgotten in the education of dentistry and dental technology in favor of modern technologies. Consider that the patient has not only lost their teeth but also a part of their identity. Yet to many in the practice of dentistry and dental technology, total prosthetics has become an annoying part of the job. This cannot continue to be the case; conditions must be created for edentulous patients that meet their individual needs for quality of life. The provision of functional full dentures must not be a privilege of prosperity.

Steffen Rohrbach, born in Germany and trained as a dental technician, was influenced early on by the philosophy of Prof Dr A. Gerber and myself, and he increasingly focused his career on solving the problem of rehabilitating the edentulous patient. After moving to the United States in 2004, for several years he worked as a clinical dental technician before joining the management team of Edmonds Dental Prosthetics in 2013. The creation of a training center for prosthetics in Springfield, Missouri, was then realized with the support of Candulor and Dr Anna Gerber in 2020.

Steffen Rohrbach's goal is to resensitize dentists and dental technology professionals to the challenges and possibilities in total prosthetics and to offer a new standard of training. In this book he records the treatment concepts that have benefitted his many patients over the years. His reflections are chronologically and extensively documented with text and excellent visual material.

This book is intended to show colleagues the way to a promising integration of individual dentures.

Peter Lerch, Prothetier SPV
Zürich, Switzerland

PREFACE

The dental rehabilitation of the fully edentulous patient has long been one of the most challenging, most distinguished, and most rewarding objectives in the fields of both dentistry and dental technology.

An overall successful rehabilitation of the edentulous patient requires both a dentist who understands how to capture all necessary data clinically and a dental laboratory technician who understands how to evaluate the gathered data and implement it into the prosthetic design. Hardly any other type of prosthetic requires such diverse skillsets from all members of the treatment team. Unlike with fixed prosthodontics, the complete denture must restore not only the patient's ability to masticate food, along with appropriate esthetics and phonetics, but also replace the hard and soft tissues lost because of atrophy. An orchestrated effort in the clinic and laboratory must include a wide range of competencies. These include comprehensive knowledge of anatomy, morphology, biology, as well as physics and mathematics. Of equal importance are excellent communication skills, tact, and intuition, along with the pertinent craftsmanship for each step.

And while our industry has made numerous efforts in the past decades to somehow simplify the process of denture-making, be it by introducing new manufacturing protocols or developing new materials, an unfortunate oversimplification has done little to improve patient care. On the contrary, patients are more than ever supplied with insufficient prosthetics, and the remaining adequately skilled clinicians and technicians are now almost considered specialists—an alarming trend that I expect will lead to a critical shortage of adequate patient care.

Personally, I had the privilege of spending my apprenticeship years in a German dental laboratory with a reputation for crafting high-end removable prosthetics. Here I learned not only how to properly fabricate complete conventional dentures but also how to design combination restorations with telescopes, including every step necessary to complete such sophisticated casework. While I also received extensive training in fixed prosthodontics, my fascination with dentures continues to this day.

In my daily work as a dental technician as well as in my role as an instructor and mentor, I attempt to raise awareness of the shortcomings of quickly produced dentures. The inadequacy of many contemporary approaches is typically the result of cost pressure in the laboratory, lack of training opportunities, and economic considerations by the treating dentist. The one who suffers is of course the patient, often unbeknownst to the treatment team, as I have found that denture patients accept even the most suboptimal solutions as an inevitable result of their tooth loss. Some of them have simply given up altogether.

It's time to change that. Our patients deserve better. Therefore, this book is intended to be a work of reference for diligent clinicians and dental technicians who want to improve patient care and deliver exceptional dentures to every patient who comes seeking their help.

Acknowledgments

My enormous gratitude goes to Quintessence Publishing for making this work possible, and to the many colleagues who encouraged me to author this book, as well as my mentors, who took a leap of faith and decided to share their own knowledge and skills with me.

This also includes the authors before me, who have inspired me over the years, first and foremost Peter Lerch, whose contributions to the field of removable prosthetics cannot be overstated. His 1986 book *Die Totale Prothetik* served as a guideline for this current work and has been a companion during my career of over 30 years. The pioneering work of Max Bosshart and Jürg Stuck should also be mentioned here in a meritorious way, as their contributions are as indispensable now as they were when first published. I am also particularly thankful to the many dentists I had the pleasure of working chairside with; without a solid understanding of their clinical procedures and challenges, my own development as a technician would not have been possible.

I also want to express my sincere appreciation to Dr Sungyong Ban, not only for his diligent review of the clinical procedures described in the following pages but also for supplementing the clinical photography. Dr Ban continues to stand out in our field with his passion, extraordinary skills, and commitment to the rehabilitation of the edentulous patient at the highest level.

Special thanks also go to my incredible team who contributed to this volume in many different ways—you guys rock! Finally, I want to thank my wife, Melissa, for her unwavering support during the creation of this work and for allowing me my "hobby" of dental technology.

"If I have seen further, it is by standing on the shoulders of giants."
—Sir Isaac Newton

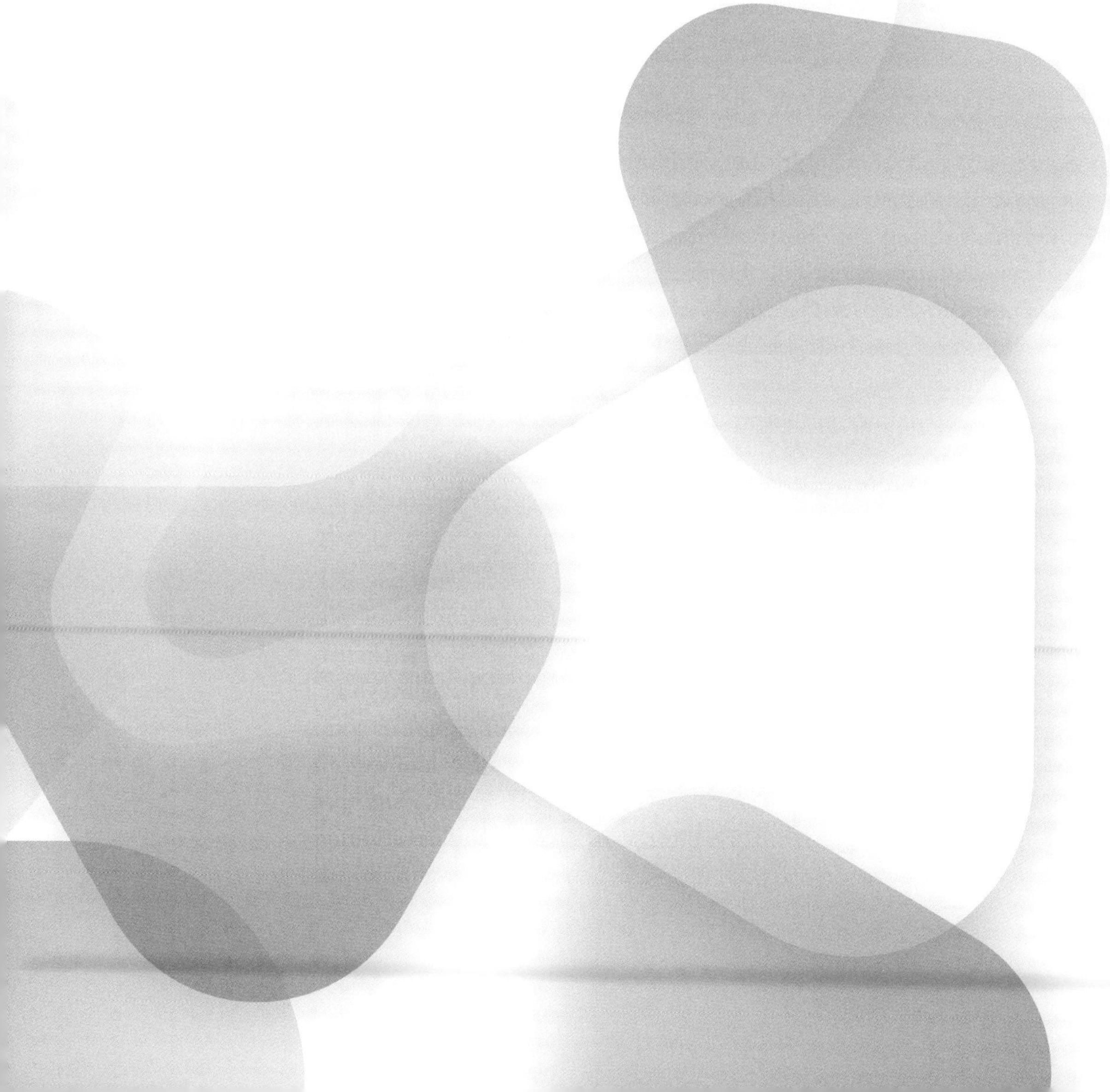

1

THE PRIMARY (ANATOMICAL) IMPRESSION

The Goal of the Primary Impression

The paramount goal of any complete, partial, or hybrid dental prosthesis is the preservation of the supporting bone, soft tissues, abutment teeth, or implants. Any form of imbalance caused by unfavorable force vectors can lead to any combination of the following:

- Discomfort, pain, and the development of repeated sore spots
- Accelerated atrophy of the residual jawbone (Fig 1-1)
- Formation of connective tissue ("flabby ridge"; Fig 1-2)
- Overgrowth of tuberosities
- Loosening of abutment teeth or implants

Unlike single-unit or most multiunit fixed prosthodontics, full-arch or removable partial restorations are connected *across* the arches, either through a denture base or a framework major connector. Therefore, we must aim for a uniform stress distribution to avoid imbalances.

The extent and shape of the denture bases, and consequently the retention, is one of the most important contributing factors to the positional stability of the prosthesis. Good positional stability achieved with a well-designed denture base will avoid or at least delay the destructive processes mentioned above. The techniques and materials used for impression taking literally lay the foundation for the prosthesis and can therefore dramatically influence case outcomes.

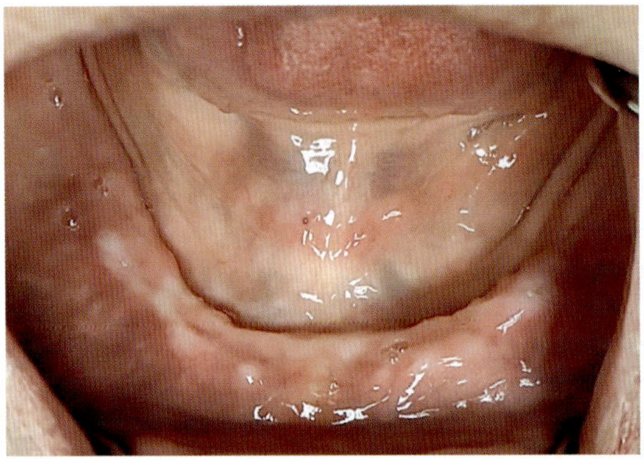

FIG 1-1 Nearly obliterated residual ridge in the mandible.

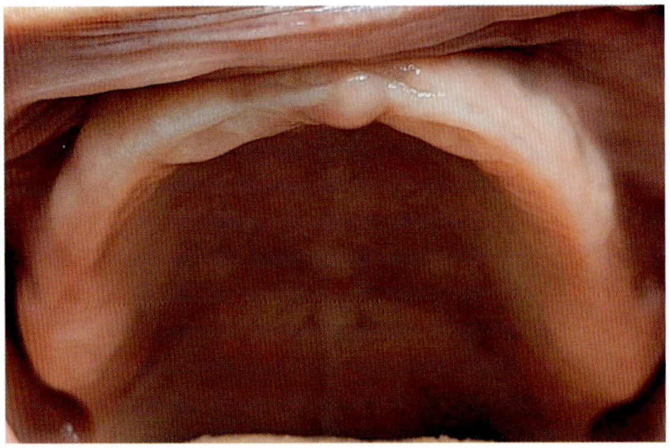

FIG 1-2 Edentulous maxilla with mild connective tissue formation in the anterior ("flabby ridge").

In general, all complete dentures and some partial dentures (altered cast technique) require a primary impression and a secondary impression. The primary impression is a deliberately overextended, static impression of the denture-bearing structures and surrounding tissues. The resulting anatomical model is used to fabricate the custom impression tray for the final functional, or myodynamic, impression.

Any subsequent steps depend on the quality of the primary impression. Missing data or defects result in more time-consuming adjustments of the custom tray and, if uncorrected, can lead to a suboptimal final model. In this scenario, inferior fit and retention of the final denture base can be expected.

Ideally, the patient should not wear any existing dental appliance for several hours prior to any impressions. A potential suction effect of the previous denture base and/or denture adhesives can lead to increased blood perfusion, which may enlarge the soft tissue. If the tissues are impressed in this engorged state, the denture fabricated will likely not fit well shortly after delivery, once the tissues recover and return to their unstressed state.

A part of the preprosthetic planning and potential treatment prior to the fabrication of any new appliance must focus on the condition of the denture-bearing structures. Any inflammation, ulceration, or other tissue pathologies should be addressed at this stage. This is of particular importance in the case of a flabby ridge (see Fig 1-2). Adapting or even relining the existing dentures can help the tissue recover and avoid the need to fabricate a new denture on potentially compressed connective tissues. A so-called "barrier reline" can also help in the treatment of denture stomatitis (thrush) in conjunction with medication treatment. Other considerations for preprosthetic treatment are discussed in chapter 4.

Maxillary primary impression

The following areas must be captured with the maxillary primary impression (see Fig 1-4):

- Complete extent of the residual alveolar ridge
- Maxillary tuberosities
- Zygomatic process
- Hamular notch/pterygomandibular fold
- Vestibular fold in an extended stage
- Labial and buccal frenula in a nondisplaced, static state
- Vibrating zone/transition area between the hard and soft palate

Mandibular primary impression

The following areas must be captured with the mandibular primary impression (see Fig 1-5):

- Complete extent of the residual alveolar ridge
- Retromolar pads
- Pterygomandibular raphe
- Sublingual and retromylohyoid areas
- Mylohyoid ridge
- Vestibular fold in an extended stage
- External oblique ridge
- Labial, lingual, and buccal frenula in a nondisplaced, static state

Selection of the Stock Tray

The selection of the stock tray influences the quality of the impression. Along with a good assortment of metal trays for edentulous arches, plastic trays are increasingly becoming the norm. Cutaway trays and thermoplastic trays are particularly useful. They can be adjusted in such a way as to not compress and distort sensitive soft tissues and structures, such as the retromolar pads.

A set of dividers can be helpful in selecting the correct width of the stock tray. In the maxilla, the buccal aspects of the tuberosities serve as a reference. In the mandible, the center points of the retromolar pads are an excellent reference. Further, the tray length must be able to support the impression material from anterior vestibule to the pterygomandibular raphe/folds. An existing denture can also be used to aid in the selection of the proper tray size.

Care must be taken to create approximately 3 mm of space in all directions to allow room for the impression material. Tissue stops can be applied with, for example, a soft silicone putty to avoid overseating of the tray during the impression. The vestibular and sublingual tray margins may be extended with compound stick, hard wax, or silicone putty. This is of particular importance in cases of advanced ridge resorption. The structures of the floor of the mouth must be prevented from prolapsing over the ridges.

Choice of Impression Material

An important goal of both primary and secondary impressions is to capture the denture bed with the soft tissues properly adapted to the underlying bone. The material of choice today is irreversible hydrocolloid (alginate). A two-viscosity system, such as AccuDent XD (Ivoclar) produces superior results (Fig 1-3). A regular alginate may be used in a similar fashion as described below, mixed in two different viscosities, with the lower viscosity loaded into a large-gauge syringe.

The material must have a consistency that allows capture of the tissue with optimal adaptation to the underlying bone, as well as adaptively extended vestibular folds and sublingual aspects. The borders of the primary impression deliberately end beyond the future prosthetic periphery to reveal all relevant landmarks and the borderline between the unattached mucosa and

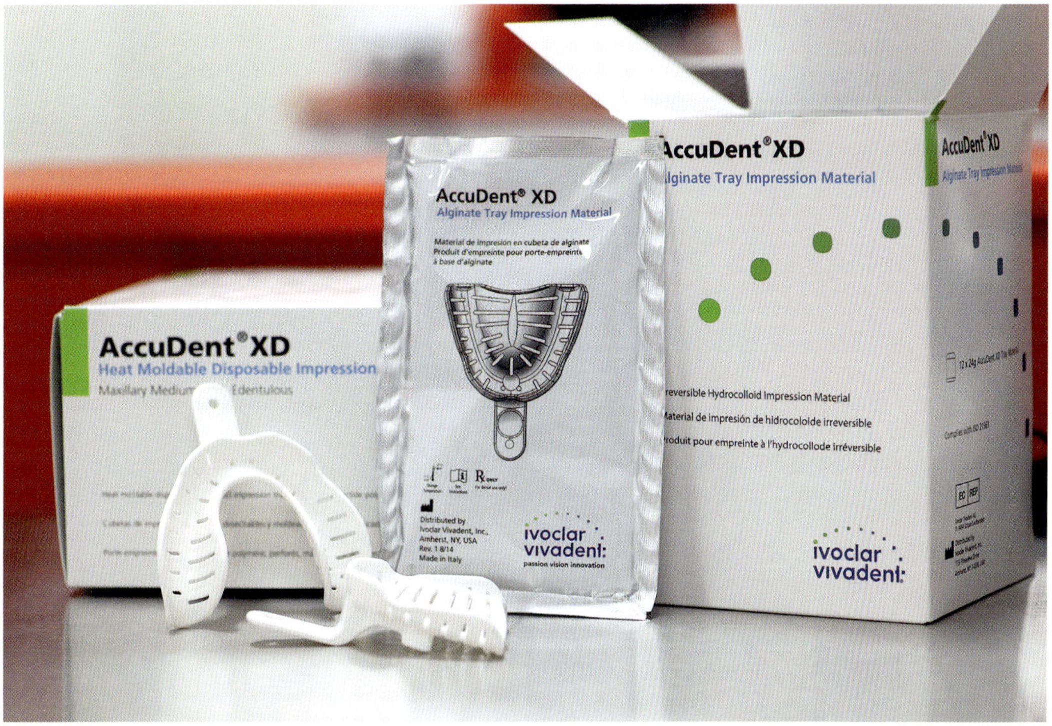

FIG 1-3 AccuDent XD with thermoplastic impression trays.

the attached gingiva, the so-called "action boundary." It must not be too dense to prevent deformation or displacement of the frenula.

Impression of the Maxilla

After the stock tray of choice has been selected and adjusted, a tray adhesive for irreversible hydrocolloids must be applied to the entire inside and outside peripheral borders of the tray. Prior to the insertion of the material into the mouth, an aspirator is used to remove saliva pools, followed by drying of the tissue with gauze. For the two-viscosity method, the low-viscosity material is mixed first and loaded into a syringe. The material is injected into the vestibule, starting from one hamular notch toward the labial frenulum. This step is then repeated on the other side. A small amount of the low-viscosity material is placed into the palatal vault. The use of retractors is recommended to prevent the loss of impression material while inserting the tray.

While the low-viscosity material is applied in the mouth, the high-viscosity component of the system is mixed, and the impression tray is loaded. The tray is then inserted into the oral cavity at a slight angle and pivoted in a rotational motion from anterior to posterior. Once the low-viscosity component previously placed in the palatal vault becomes visible at the dorsal portion of the impression, the tray is held in place.

With the impression remaining in place, the clinician shapes the anterior vestibule by placing the index finger and thumb to the left and right of the philtrum, gently moving the upper lip inferiorly. The buccal vestibule is shaped in a similar fashion by gently moving the cheeks in a rotating and downward motion.

Once the material is set, the impression is removed and checked for any voids or defects (Fig 1-4).

Impression of the Mandible

The preparation of the tray for the mandible is analogous to the maxilla, as described above. The sublingual borders of the tray must be checked once more to ensure that the sublingual glands are prevented from prolapsing onto the posterior ridge.

The low-viscosity component is mixed and loaded into a syringe and injected from one retromolar pad to the labial frenulum. This is repeated on the other side before the tray loaded with the high-viscosity component is inserted into the oral cavity. Again, the use of retractors is recommended. For the impression of the mandible, the tray is seated first around the retromolar pads and then pivoted toward the anterior vestibule. Great care must be taken not to compress or distort the retromolar pads and pterygomandibular ligaments by applying excessive pressure.

Once the material is set, the impression is removed and checked for any voids or defects (Fig 1-5).

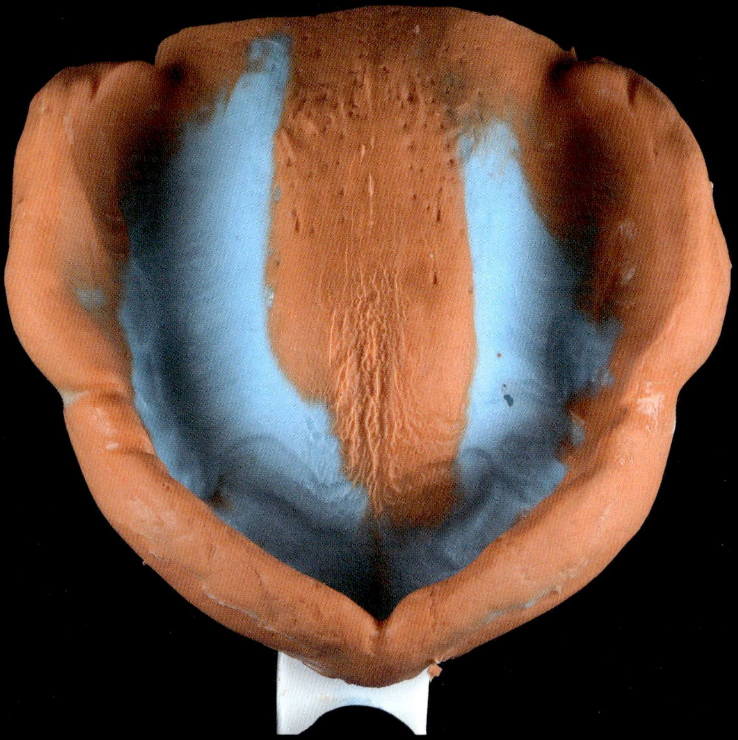

FIG 1-4 Preliminary impression of the maxilla.

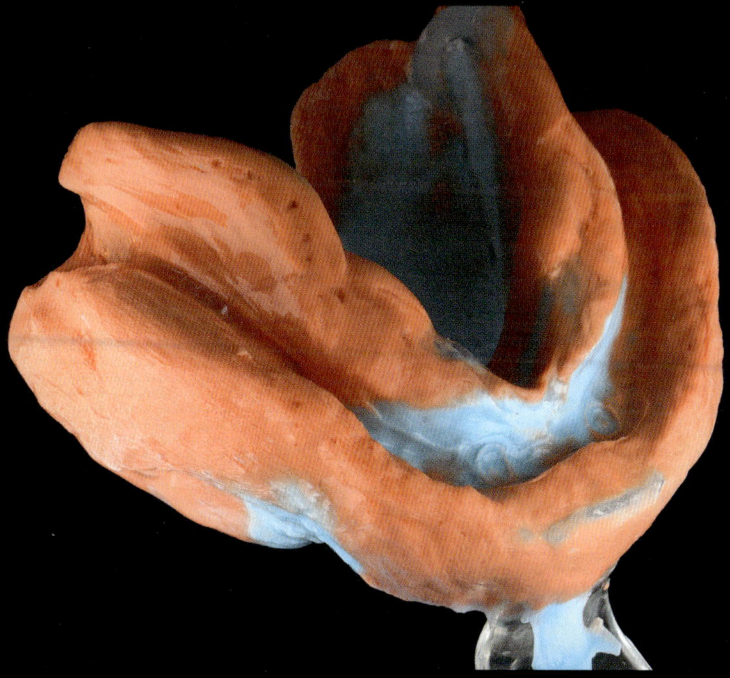

FIG 1-5 Preliminary impression of the mandible.

Disinfection

After the impressions are completed, they are rinsed under cold running water and disinfected. The disinfectant manufacturer's instructions for use must be strictly followed to avoid contamination with any potential infectious material. Irreversible hydrocolloid is to be poured immediately. However, dimensional stability and storage times differ from one system to another.

The Anatomical Model

Safety always comes first. As such, all materials and impressions received from the dental office must be disinfected upon arrival at the laboratory. The impression should be dabbed with tissue to remove water or pools of disinfectant. Compressed air should not be used because it could introduce potentially infectious material into the air and damage the delicate alginate material.

For the fabrication of the anatomical model, an ISO Type 3 gypsum stone is recommended. The stone powder and the water must be measured diligently and ideally mixed under vacuum. The manufacturer's instructions for use will show the powder-to-water ratio, along with soaking, stirring, and setting times. The use of a model base former is highly recommended. This will save material and time when trimming the models.

In general, light vibration should be used when pouring the impressions to avoid air bubble inclusion. The maxillary impression is best poured by placing a small amount of stone onto the highest point of the palatal vault. The stone then flows into the alveolar ridge. For the mandibular impression, it is best to place a small amount of stone into one retromolar pad area and guide the stone through the alveolar ridge toward the other side.

When the impression is filled, it should be placed away from the vibrating table to avoid spilling while pouring the base. A wall-mounted bracket can be useful here. The primary impressions are then inverted onto the prepared stone base. Building up small mounds of stone dorsal to the retromolar pads helps to prevent breakage of the model heels during later steps.

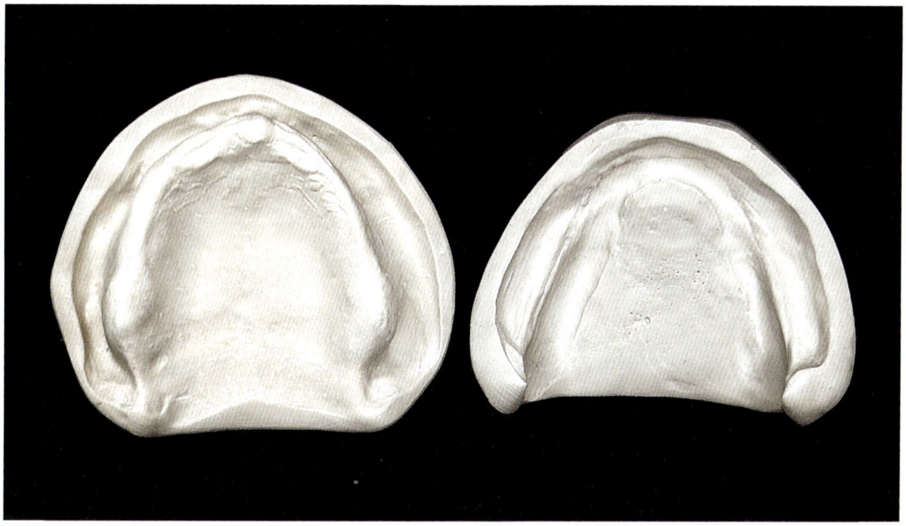

FIG 1-6 Anatomical models from preliminary impressions.

Once the stone has completely set, the impression tray is removed, and the model is inspected (Fig 1-6). Any small beads are cleared. Before trimming the model base, it can be helpful to mark the periphery; this prevents accidental overtrimming. A uniform, 2- to 3-mm-wide model margin is to be created. The underside of the model should be parallel to the alveolar ridge and at a right angle to the sides of the model.

2

THE FUNCTIONAL IMPRESSION TRAY

The secondary, myofunctional (myodynamic) impression with an intelligently designed custom impression tray creates the definitive basis for the final restoration. It is the only reliable method to ensure excellent superimposition of the intaglio surfaces onto the denture-bearing structures and to establish the peripheral valve margins (see next section). Perfect fit and an optimal suction effect secures the dentures during everyday activities such as chewing, speaking, singing, kissing, laughing, etc.

Frequently, this crucial step of the myofunctional impression is omitted for the perceived benefit of saving time and cost. In this case, the overextended anatomical model is used to create record bases and the final denture. The shortcomings of this approach cannot be overstated. The omission of the secondary impression inevitably leads to time-consuming adjustments of the record bases and the final dentures. Further, an ill-fitting base may result in inaccurate records and subsequent remounts and resets. During the finishing steps of the fabrication process, the dental laboratory technician will have to "guess" the border length, thickness, and contours. It is not uncommon that the prosthesis needs to be relined after multiple unsuccessful attempts at border adjustments. Therefore, this approach not only results in suboptimal patient care but is also economically unsound.

The Valve Margin

Achieving retention of the maxillary and even the mandibular complete denture relies on establishing a so-called "valve margin" during the functional impression. The term describes a continuous peripheral border of the dentures, including the postpalatal seal in the maxilla, which creates a hermetic seal between the intaglio surface of the dentures and the oral mucosa. The myofunctional impression records the length and thickness of these margins by means of border molding. Myodynamic movements in the areas of the mucogingival boundary ("action-boundary"), the sublingual musculature, and the frenula attachments are recorded in this step. Compared to the anatomical impression, this will show only the areas of the denture bed that are not affected by movements. When established correctly and maintained in the final denture borders, the valve margin seals in a sufficient amount of saliva and prevents air or food from entering under the dentures. The valve margin consists of an inner valve, which lies against the action boundary on the intaglio surface, and an outer valve, which adapts to the mucosa of the lip and cheek in the vestibular fornix.

The goal of the valve margin is therefore to take advantage of several physical effects that help prevent the dentures from lifting during function:

- An atmospheric effect through a continuous airtight seal
- Adhesion acting between saliva and the intaglio surface
- Cohesion acting within the saliva film

Materials for the Custom Tray

Several materials are commonly used for the fabrication of the custom impression tray:

- Light-curing resin sheets
- Thermoplastics for vacuum forming
- Self-curing resins

The main drawback of light-curing resins is their unreliable dimensional stability. Even with diligent adaptation to the model, one can easily observe the changes that occur during polymerization. This becomes evident with

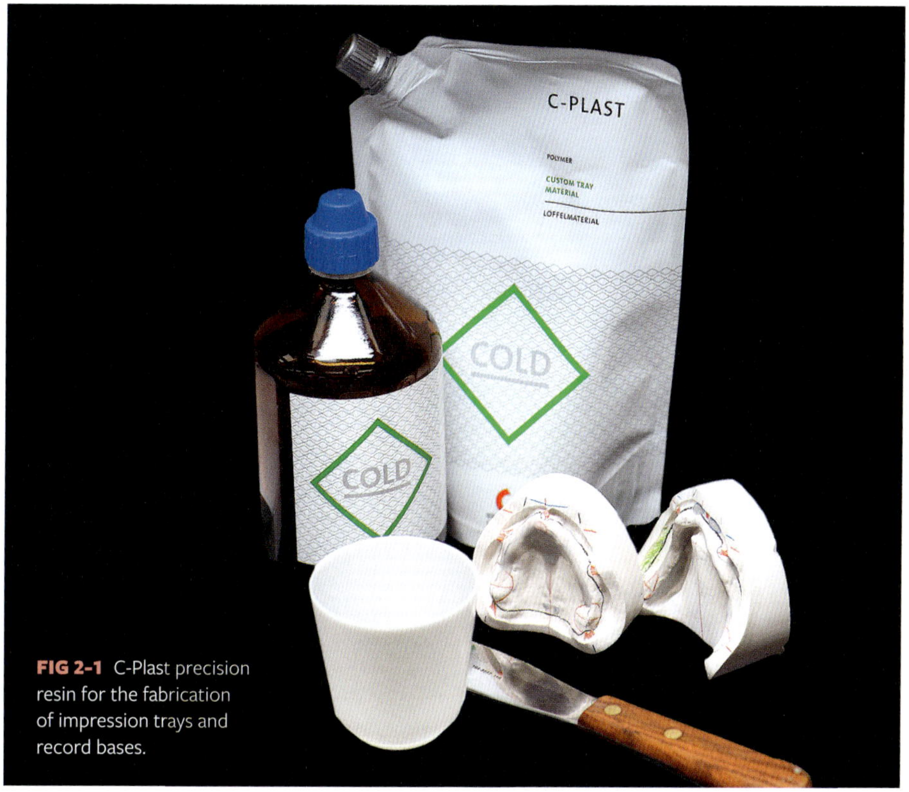

FIG 2-1 C-Plast precision resin for the fabrication of impression trays and record bases.

gaps forming at the dorsal margins of the palate and tighter-than-intended areas like the buccal surfaces of the maxillary tuberosities. Vacuum-formed thermoplastics are also problematic because they tend to flex and subsequently distort during the creation of the functional impression. Due to the vacuum-forming process, the critical vestibular and sublingual borders are often too short and ill-adapted.

The logical choice is an autopolymerizing resin like C-Plast (Candulor; Fig 2-1). It is a dimensionally stable material with virtually no shrinkage. Unlike light-curing resins, autopolymerizing resins do not contain silica and are therefore easier and safer to work with, and they generally do not dull carbide burs. These self-curing resins are available as a polymer/monomer kit.

The Myostatic Outline

The model produced from the primary impression defines the anatomical characteristics of the denture-bearing areas. The peripheral borders are impressed passively overextended; that is, they do not take the muscular freeway space into account. To create a functional tray suitable for border molding, a myostatic outline is created. In the first step, the following structures are identified and marked with a pencil:

- In the maxilla:
  - Maxillary tuberosities
  - Incisive papilla
  - Labial and buccal frenula
  - Pterygomandibular ligament
  - Vibrating zone

- In the mandible:
  - Retromolar pads
  - Someya sinew string, if present
  - Buccal border of the external oblique ridge
  - Mylohyoid ridge
  - Lingual, labial, and buccal frenula

The markings of the relevant landmarks are then connected by a line that will define the peripheral borders of the tray (Fig 2-2). This line should run about 3 mm short from the lowest point of the vestibular fold (Fig 2-3). Sublingually, it should stop right at the mylohyoid ridge, or slightly short of it (Fig 2-4). It is important to fully encompass the maxillary tuberosities and the retromolar pads. The latter should be inspected closely: the buccal margins of the retromolar pads should not be exceeded, as fibers of the masseter muscle insert in this area. According to Abe, in about 15% to 20% of patients, the Someya sinew string can be identified, and it must be avoided. The external

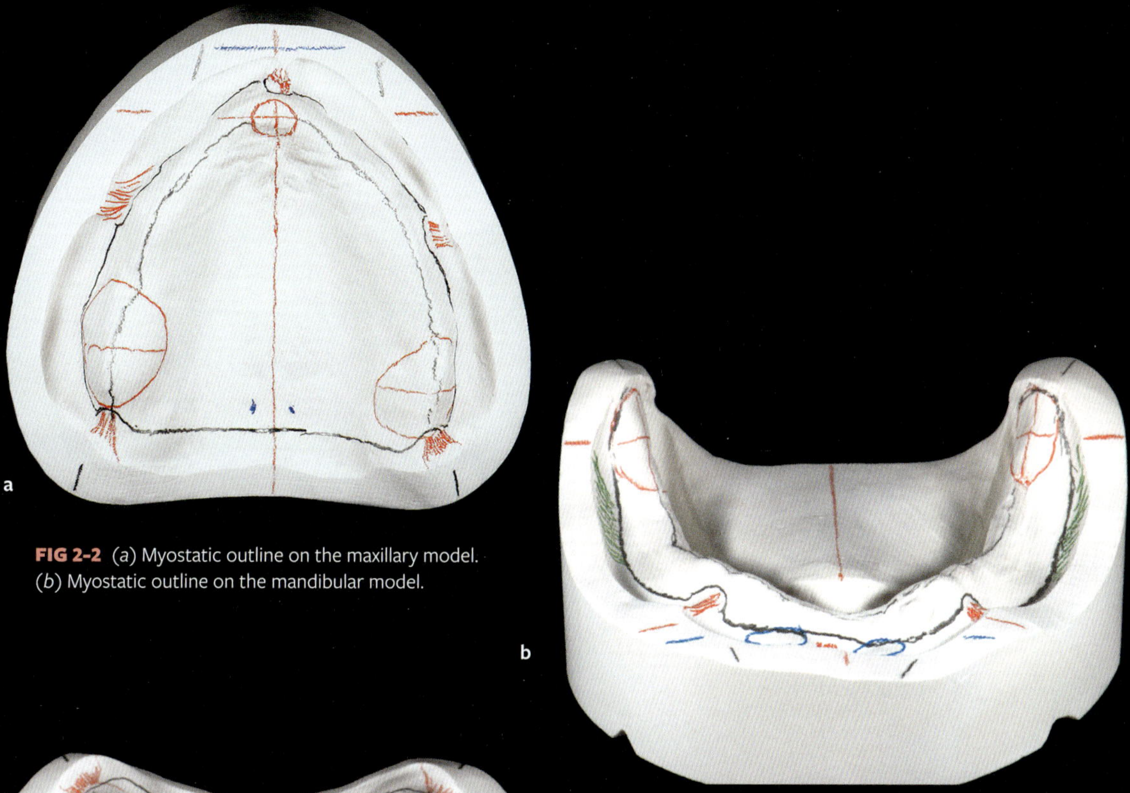

a

b

FIG 2-2 (*a*) Myostatic outline on the maxillary model. (*b*) Myostatic outline on the mandibular model.

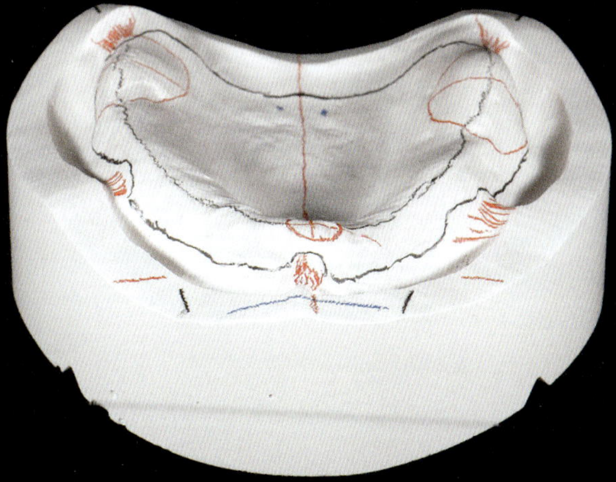

FIG 2-3 The border length of the tray should be approximately 3 mm shorter than the vestibular fold.

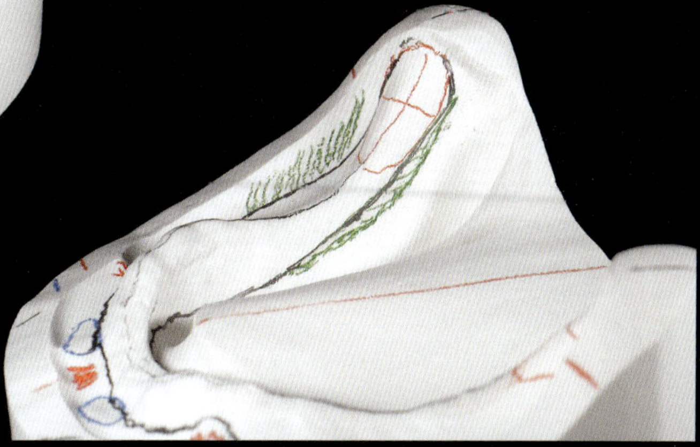

FIG 2-4 The paralingual margins should be approximately 1 mm shorter than the myohyoid line.

oblique ridge has enormous potential for creating positional stability, as it is an anatomical feature that is little affected by atrophy. However, caution is advised to not extend the border too far buccally, as fibers of the buccinator muscle insert into this area. All frenula must be generously avoided to create the necessary freeway space during the dynamic impression.

It is important to understand that the final valve margins are established by the material chosen for border molding and not by the tray margins themselves. Therefore, it can be said that the tray margins serve as a carrier for the impression material.

Model Preparation

Before the fabrication of the custom tray, the model must be blocked out with wax. This step serves two purposes: *(1)* It prevents pressure in sensitive areas, and *(2)* it avoids damage to the model in undercut areas. The traditional approach of covering the entire anatomical part of the model with a layer of baseplate wax leads to a "floating" impression tray and is therefore advised against. The creation of tissue stops in custom trays by cutting small "windows" into the blockout layer is controversial, as they often lead to tissue compressions during the impression, later clearly visible as dimples in the master models.

The pressure-sensitive areas of concern in the maxilla are the incisive papilla, the palatal rugae, the median suture, the fovea palatinae, and any potential palatal tori (Fig 2-5). In the mandible, the mentalis muscle attachments and the region of the mental foramen should be blocked out with wax (Fig 2-6). In both arches, the crest of the residual ridge should also be covered by a thin layer of wax. This is particularly important in the mandible, as a small band of connective tissue can often be found on a very resorbed ridge crest, which is extremely sensitive to pressure.

After the model is sufficiently blocked out, it should be soaked for 15 minutes in lukewarm water to eliminate air on the stone surface. The warm model should then be dried gently, and an alginate-based separating agent such as Iso-K (Candulor; Fig 2-7) should be applied with a clean, soft paintbrush that has been lightly dampened with water. Pooling of the separator needs to be avoided, especially in the vestibules and the paratubic (buccal of the maxillary tuberosities) and sublingual areas. Once the first layer has set, a second thin coat

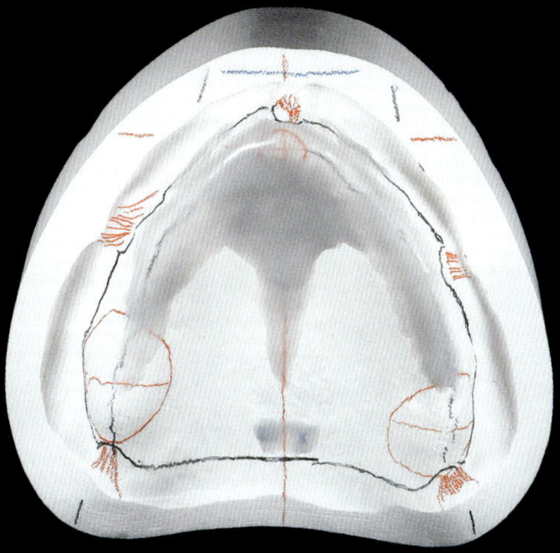

FIG 2-5 Blockout of the maxilla includes the incisive papilla, the palatal rugae, the fovea palatinae, and the crest of the ridge.

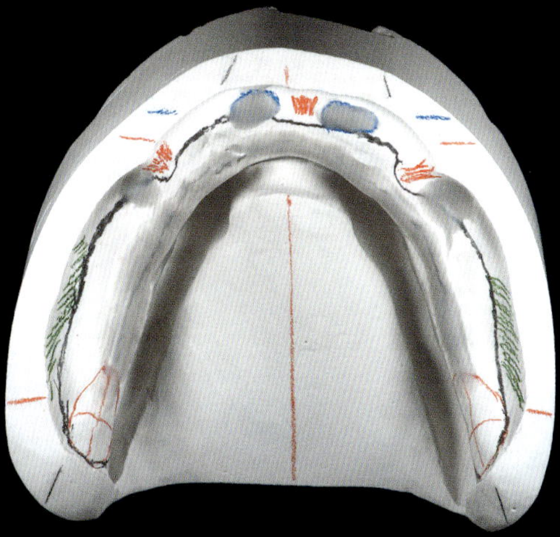

FIG 2-6 Blockout of the mandible includes the mentalis muscle attachments, the mental foramina, and the crest of the ridge.

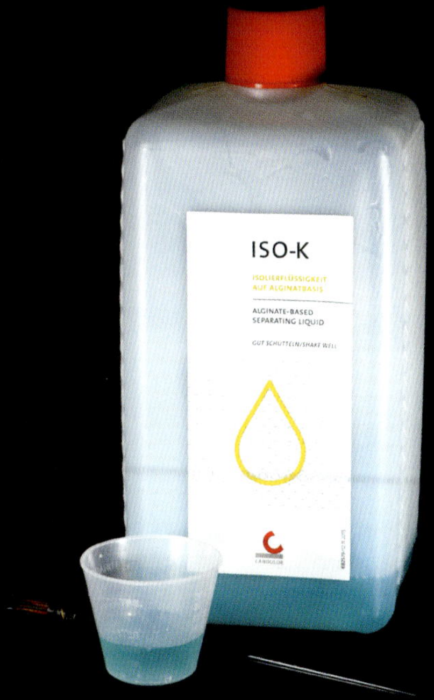

FIG 2-7 An alginate-based separating agent is best suited to insulate the watered models against resin.

may be applied. Depending on the ambient temperature, the separator will dry completely in about 15 minutes.

Tray Designs

The most common design for the functional impression tray features a handle that is attached to the base and protrudes past the lips at approximately a 90-degree angle. The drawback of this design is that the anterior vestibule is not impressed in a myofunctional state but is distorted by the handle. In addition to this disadvantage, the pressure exerted onto the denture-bearing areas originates from an unphysiologic angle and is arbitrarily dictated by the clinician. As mentioned in the previous chapter, the aim must be for a uniform stress distribution and tissue adaptation to avoid imbalances under masticatory function.

It thus seems logical to dispense with the use of protruding handles altogether. Remarkable success can be achieved with the closed-mouth technique. Instead of traditional handles, resin bars in the shape similar to a wax rim are created. This design allows the clinician to take the impressions with the bars of the maxillary and mandibular trays occluding to capture the borders and denture-bearing tissues in the same state as when the final denture is used during mastication. This technique is described in detail in chapter 3.

As already mentioned, the same parameters of a standardized wax rim are used to design the resin bars: The anterior height of the rim measures 20 to 22 mm in the maxilla and 16 to 18 mm in the mandible from the anterior vestibule to the "incisal" edge (Fig 2-8). Transverse and sagittal planes can be established with the aid of a rim former. If a preliminary bite record is available, the bars can be accurately fabricated in the articulator, ensuring parallelism between the occlusal surfaces of the bars.

Special consideration must be given to cases presenting with structural changes similar to combination syndrome (ie, edentulous maxilla and partially edentulous mandible with only anterior teeth remaining). To avoid a deformed

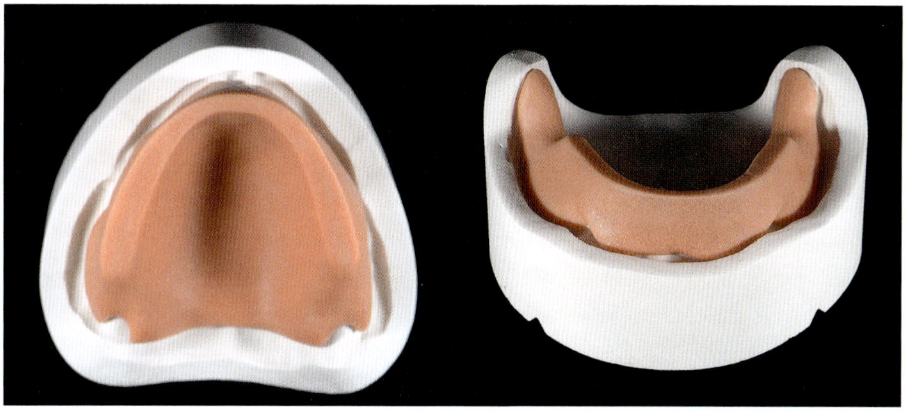

FIG 2-8 The contours of the impression trays for the closed-mouth technique follow the same principles as the standardized wax rim.

impression of the connective tissue that is often found in the anterior maxilla (flabby ridge), a windowed tray design can be advantageous. Here, an opening is created in the area marked by the dentist. The impression is first taken in a conventional fashion. Using a scalpel or a similar instrument, the area of the flabby ridge is then cut out of the impression. After the tray is reinserted, the connective tissue will show in an uncompressed state through this window. As a last step, the area is covered with a low-viscosity material such as a light-bodied polyvinyl siloxane.

Fabrication of the Functional Impression Tray

Once the separating agent is fully dried, the tray resin material is mixed according to the manufacturer's instructions for use. The resulting resin dough is smooth and pliable and can be shaped for about 5 to 7 minutes. The base and the bars can be fabricated at the same time or in stages, depending on experience. The dough can be applied directly to the model or placed onto

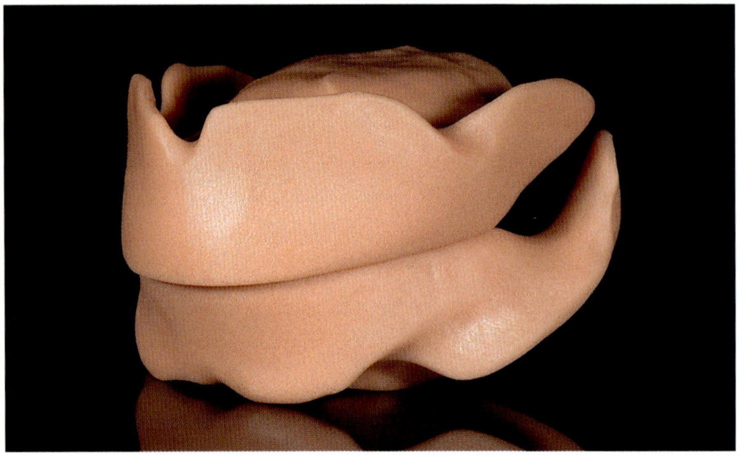

FIG 2-9 The myofunctional trays are designed to occlude without any interference. Adaptive spaces for the perioral musculature are created.

a working surface and formed into sheets with a small silicone-coated rolling pin. Alternatively, the material can be formed into a roll of about half an inch. The roll is then placed onto the crest of the ridge and, using the thumb and index finger, shaped into the periphery and the palate. Gloves should be worn when working with uncured PMMA-based materials.

The best density of the material can be achieved by placing the tray into a water-filled pressurized curing unit at 2 bar and 40°C for 7 minutes; however, the material will also polymerize on the bench. After the material is fully polymerized, the tray is removed from the model and shaped with conventional carbide burs. Final smoothing can be easily achieved with rotating sandpaper strips. The border length should follow the previously drawn myostatic outline precisely, and adaptive spaces for the perioral musculature should be created (Fig 2-9). After a final control and thorough cleaning in an ultrasonic unit, the trays are ready for submission to the dentist.

3

THE MYOFUNCTIONAL IMPRESSION

The purpose of the myofunctional impression is to accurately reproduce the attached gingiva, ensuring a tight fit of the inner valves. It records the freeway space of the frenula and perioral musculature to accurately capture the extent, contour, and course of the peripheral borders. By doing so, it enables a gap-free attachment to the cheek and lip, allowing for a seamless impression of the inner and outer valve margins.

Another important aspect of the myofunctional impression is the representation of the vibration zone. In conjunction with the later etching of the post-dam (or postpalatal seal), this helps create a tight dorsal seal, ensuring a secure fit of the denture. Additionally, the myofunctional impression plays a vital role in the positioning of the tongue. It allows for the greatest possible freedom of movement for the tongue, without it becoming an opponent of the denture. This positioning also supports the later acceptance of the denture in the mandible, promoting comfort and functionality for the patient.

Preparation for the Myofunctional Impression

Regardless of the chosen design of the impression tray, the first step is to inspect the border length of the tray in situ. After a visual check, the patient is asked to open and close the mouth, producing sounds like "aaah," "eeeh," and "oooh"; placing their tongue over the anterior part of the mandibular tray; and pushing their tongue into the left and right cheeks. The patient also performs grimaces and is instructed to move the mandible from side to side. During each of these test movements, the clinician must observe and correct any lifting or dislodgement of the tray through selective grinding with a carbide bur.

In the maxilla, the most corrections can be expected in the areas of the tuberosities, due to excessive thickness of the tray material. The distobuccal aspect of the tuberosities is often narrowed by the transverse movement of the coronoid processes of the mandible.

In the mandible, corrections are to be expected buccal of the retromolar pads, where the fibers of the masseter muscle insert, sublingually around the mylohyoid ridge, and in the labial vestibule.

An effective method for checking border interference consists of using a light-bodied polyvinyl siloxane (PVS) around the functional margins. After insertion into the mouth, the test movements described above are followed by the patient sucking on the clinician's index finger. After the material has set, the tray is removed from the mouth and any overextension is revealed by tray-burn or press-through. These areas can now be easily adjusted in length and/or width with a carbide bur.

If the closed-mouth technique is used, an occlusal adjustment on the bars of the custom impression trays may be necessary. During the impressions, the patient must be able to exert even pressure onto the bars of the trays.

Choice of Material for the Myofunctional Impression

In the author's experience, good technique is more important than the choice of material. Superior results are usually achieved with a two-phase approach, in which the functional borders are created in the first step and the definitive impression in a second step. Some common choices to establish the functional borders include polyether, such as Impregum (3M); suspension polymer plasters, such as Softone (Keystone Industries); heavy-body PVS, such as HoneyGum Rigid Extra Fast (DMG); or thermoplastics, such as Iso-Functional (GC America) or Kerr Impression Compound (Kerr Dental).

The definitive impression is completed subsequently, typically with a light-body PVS.

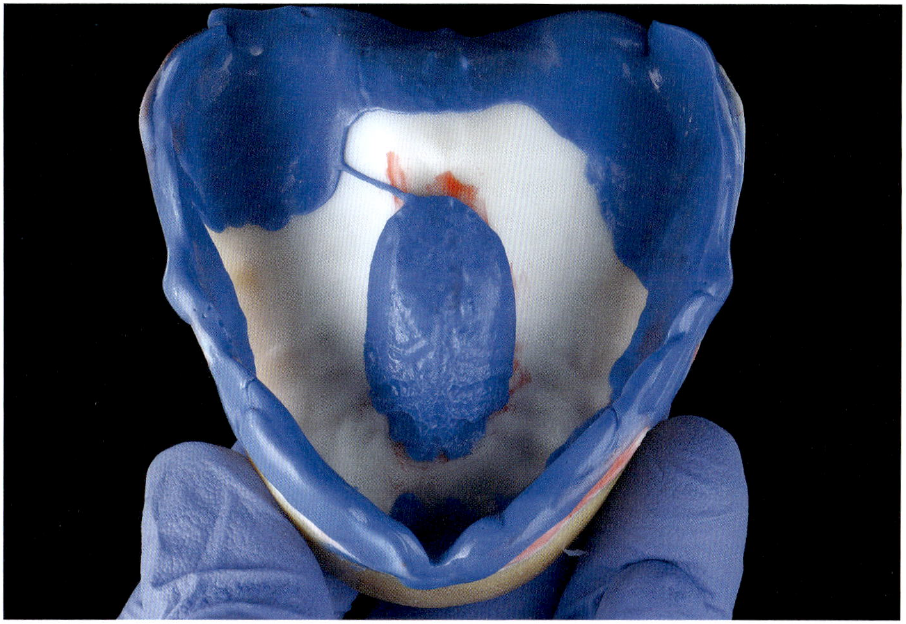

FIG 3-1 Border-molded maxillary impression.

Example Sequence for the Closed-Mouth Technique

While the choice of impression material and technique falls under the clinician's competence, a suggested sequence of steps for the closed-mouth impression technique using a combination of PVS materials with different viscosities is listed below.

For the maxilla

1. Tray adhesive is applied exclusively on the borders of the tray. This ensures the retention of the impression material during all subsequent steps.
2. Heavy-body PVS is then applied solely to the borders of the tray. This viscous material helps establish the functional borders, or valve margins, of the final denture base (Fig 3-1).
3. The tray is gently inserted into the patient's mouth, and its position is initially stabilized by the clinician's index finger on the palate. This

provides a secure anchor point and prevents any movement of the tray during the impression process.

4. The patient is instructed to perform a sucking motion on the clinician's index finger multiple times, alternating with short periods of muscle relaxation. This action helps create a uniform pressure distribution within the oral cavity, aiding in the accurate capture of the mucostatic areas.
5. The patient is asked to open their mouth and move their mandible from side to side a few times, all while maintaining an open position. This lateral movement helps create the functional space needed by the coronoid process. The patient is finally instructed to open the mouth wide and close, alternating a few times, until the material sets. Ideally, the functional impression should exhibit significant suction upon removal, indicating proper establishment of the inner and outer valve margin.
6. Once the impression is removed, any excess material on the dorsal area of the impression is trimmed if needed. This step prevents any triggering of the gag reflex during the next stages.
7. The remaining surfaces of the tray are thoroughly dried, and tray adhesive is applied.
8. A thin layer of light-body PVS is then applied to the remaining surfaces of the tray. This fluid material effectively captures the detailed features of the mucosa, ensuring a precise impression for the optimal superimposition of the future denture base.
9. The tray is reinserted into the patient's mouth, and any excess material on the dorsal area is removed using a dental mirror or a large aspirator. **IMPORTANT:** At this stage the patient is asked to repeat the previous movements to prevent the wash material from flowing into established freeway spaces. This ensures the integrity and accuracy of the border impression.
10. Once the second phase of the maxillary impression is completed, the tray is removed. A significant amount of suction should be observed. Any remaining dorsal excess is trimmed.

If any uncertainty arises regarding the quality of the impression, rinsing the impression with water, careful inspection, and reinsertion can provide further assurance of a sufficient suction effect. Figure 3-2 shows a completed myofunctional impression of the maxilla.

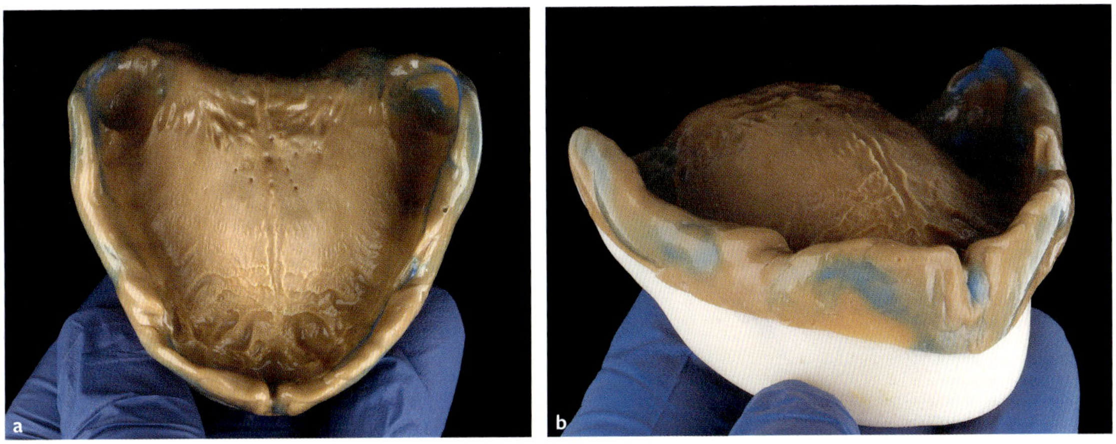

FIG 3-2 (*a*) Completed myofunctional impression with PVS. (*b*) The inner and outer valve margins are established.

For the mandible

1. The process begins by carefully reinserting the maxillary tray into the patient's oral cavity, ensuring a proper fit. Tray adhesive is applied only along the borders of the mandibular tray. It is recommended to apply petroleum jelly or a similar material around the distobuccal area of the maxillary impression, because material from the mandibular arch may adhere to the maxillary impression.
2. Next, heavy-body PVS material is applied exclusively to the borders of the tray, similar to the first step of the maxillary impression (Fig 3-3).
3. With the tray securely in place, the patient is given specific instructions to follow. The patient is asked to alternate between biting down firmly onto the occluding bars and relaxing. Then they are instructed to pout their lips, producing an "oooooooh" sound, followed by a smile that creates an "eeeeeeeh" sound. This is repeated two to three times, before the patient is directed to wet their upper lip.
4. Further instructions are given to the patient, involving tongue movements from left to right, which helps to capture the sublingual muscle activity. The patient is then instructed to swallow. These movements are repeated two to three times.

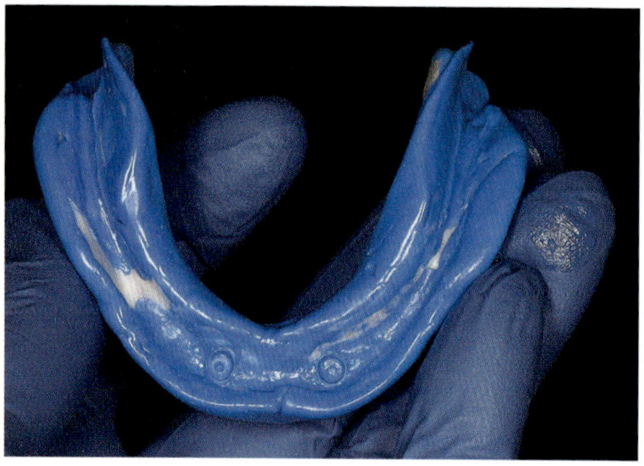

FIG 3-3 Border-molded impression of the mandible.

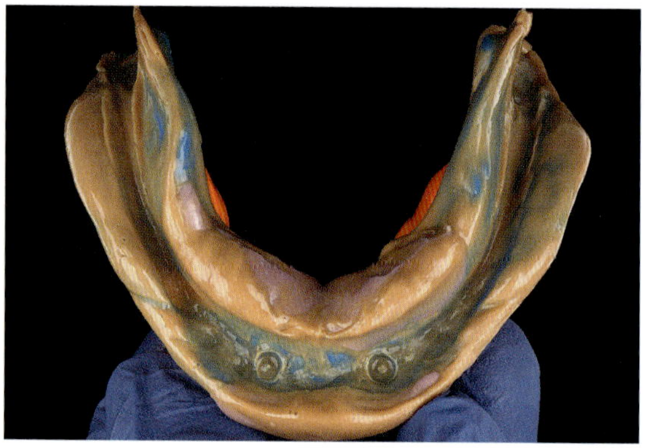

FIG 3-4 Completed myofunctional impression of the mandible (here with healing abutments of two implants). The sublingual area has been further enhanced with putty to create a sublingual roll.

5. Once the initial impression is complete, the tray is removed, and the PVS material and the tray's intaglio surface are carefully dried. Tray adhesive is then applied to the remaining surfaces of the tray. It is vital to control the application of light-body PVS material, as it is thinly layered onto the tray, enhancing the accuracy of the impression.
6. The tray is then reinserted into the patient's mouth, repeating the previous movements to prevent the light-body PVS material from flowing into the established freeway spaces. When the setting time has elapsed, the mandibular tray is removed. Ideally, a suction effect is evident during this removal process. Finally, any excess material on the tray, particularly along the dorsal area, is carefully trimmed if necessary.

Figure 3-4 shows a completed myofunctional impression of the mandible.

After the impressions are completed, they are rinsed under cold running water and disinfected. The disinfectant manufacturer's instruction for use must be strictly followed to avoid contamination with any potential infectious material.

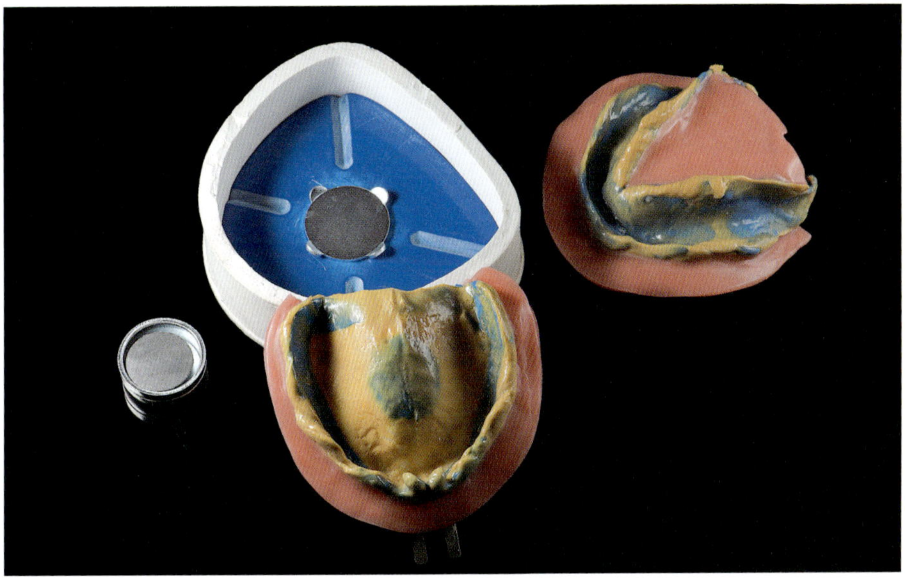

FIG 3-5 Beaded myofunctional impressions ready for pouring.

Master Model Fabrication

In order to preserve the established functional borders of the impression, the technician must choose one of two methods: beading or boxing.

To prepare for model fabrication with the beading method, the technician will add a strip of baseplate wax or beading wax about 3 mm above the impression borders (Fig 3-5). It is recommended to add a very thin layer of hot wax to the area before beading wax is applied. Additionally, the lingual area is blocked out with a piece of baseplate wax to avoid time-consuming grinding later on. The use of a base former, such as the Pin-Cast Model base former (Renfert), is strongly recommended.

The boxing method presupposes either the use of baseplate wax, a magnetic strip, or a boxing system like the SAM Magnetic Split Cast Former (SAM

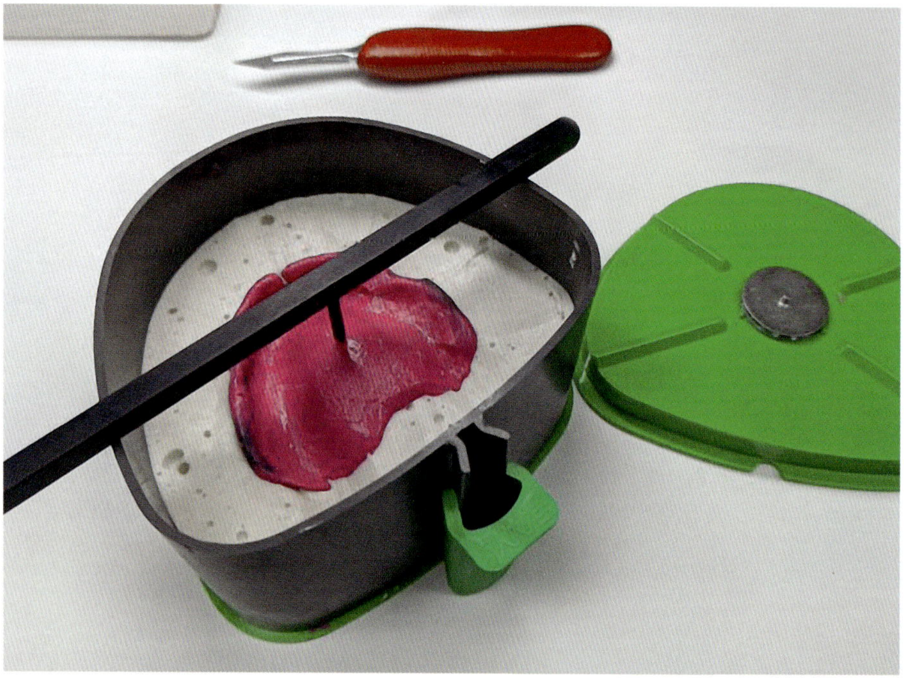

FIG 3-6 Boxing of the myofunctional impression using the SAM Magnetic Split Cast Former.

Präzisionstechnik; Fig 3-6). Here the impression is placed into a soft medium such as modeling compound, alginate, or a mixture of pumice and plaster held by a ring.

Regardless of the method used, the inclusion of a magnet and counter plate, along with a split cast, is helpful. This way the model will later accurately set back into the articulator for the purpose of the laboratory remount, without the messy use of glue or sticky wax. It also makes handling the models during setting and waxing much more convenient.

For the fabrication of the final myofunctional model, an ISO Type 4 natural stone is recommended. If an injection protocol is used for processing, an ISO Type 3 will be sufficient. Synthetic or semisynthetic resin-reinforced stones are not indicated in combination with PMMA processing.

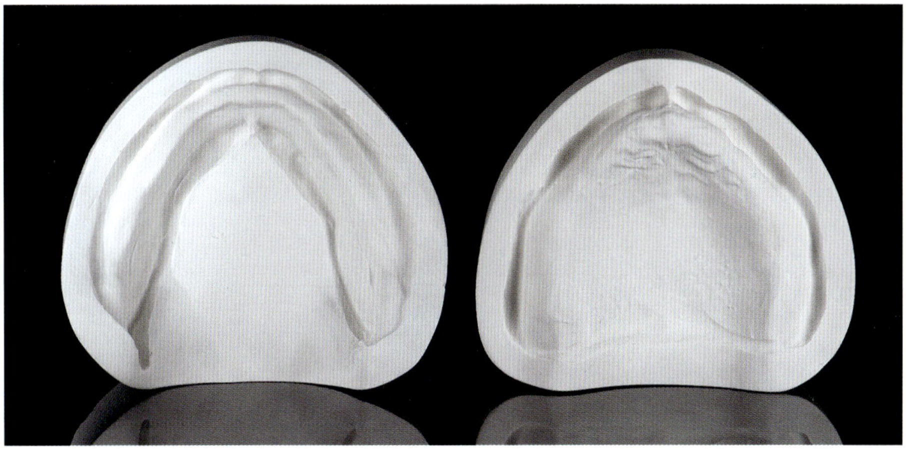

FIG 3-7 Final master models with 3- to 4-mm-wide model margins.

The fully set model is freed from the impression tray and any remaining impression material before trimming. Small beads are carefully removed. The model margins are to be 3 to 4 mm wide, and the sides of the model must be at a right angle to the base (Fig 3-7). Finishing the nonanatomical parts of the model with a wet sandpaper strip makes for a neat presentation and makes later model analysis easier.

Conclusion

The sequence shown previously in this chapter is only one of several techniques. Ultimately, the method chosen lies within the competence of the clinician.

Regardless of the technique used, diligence and following the correct instructions and steps are paramount to capturing an accurate and suction-effective impression. Adherence to a systematic sequence of steps ensures a meticulous and clinically appropriate workflow that with time will become second nature, resulting in an accurate and reliable record of the myostatic areas of the denture-bearing structures.

4

REGISTRATION

Physiologic Centric Relation

The determination of the vertical and horizontal relationship between the maxillary and mandibular arches is an essential step in the fabrication of any full-arch rehabilitation. The goal here is to create an accurate record of the physiologic centric relation between the condyles and the glenoid fossae.

In natural dentition, a discrepancy between maximal intercuspation (MIP, also known as *habitual intercuspation*), and centric occlusion is not uncommon and of little consequence. In conventional dentures, however, the aim is to create a situation where centric occlusion and MIP are identical. Any significant incongruity forces the patient to "search for" MIP and thereby likely glide over the inclined ridges of the occlusal surfaces. This can lead to small tipping movements of the denture body, subsequently creating repeated sore spots, and must therefore be avoided.

The most recent *Glossary of Prosthodontic Terms* (GPT-9) defines *centric relation* as the following:

> A maxillomandibular relationship, independent of tooth contact, in which the condyles articulate in the anterior-superior position against the posterior slopes of the articular eminences; in this position, the mandible is restricted to a purely rotary movement; from this unstrained, physiologic, maxillo-mandibular relationship, the patient can make vertical, lateral, or protrusive movements; it is a clinically useful, repeatable reference position."

Gerber similarly described this as "the pressure-less, physiological zenith position," which is easily reproducible.

It is important to understand that centric relation varies depending on the vertical distance between the jaws. Thus, an accurate record of centric relation must be obtained at the correct vertical dimension of occlusion (VDO). Determining the correct VDO also has far-reaching consequences for the orofacial appearance of the patient, and ultimately masticatory and phonetic function.

Capturing physiologic centric relation and VDO is not always a simple task for the clinician. Countless approaches have been researched and used, and many are meritorious in their own right.

Neuromuscular Programming

Gerber's extensive research has shown the interrelation between the stomatognathic system and individual neuromuscular programming. He described a form of feedback loop, with the central nervous system (CNS) as the controlling element. The CNS constantly receives sensory information from the nerves of the teeth, the masticatory musculature, the periodontal apparatus, and the tissues of the temporomandibular joint (TMJ). In turn, the CNS develops a pattern that controls masticatory movements and guides the mandible into MIP position.

Preprosthetic Treatment

Patients presenting with existing complete dentures frequently show a diminished VDO due to abrasive wear of the posterior prosthetic teeth. Over time, this loss of vertical dimension leads to a pseudoprognathic position along with habitual mastication in the anterior region. As a consequence, the neuromuscular programming is altered, as are the length and flexibility of the masticatory musculature. If this pathologic state is not addressed, a new set of dentures is likely to copy these pathologies.

One approach to return the stomatognathic system to a physiologic state is the restoration of VDO through a buildup of the existing dentures, similar to the preparation of an occlusal splint. Depending on the severity of the collapsed VDO, this measure can be completed either chairside with the addition of direct composite or tooth-colored acrylic or in the laboratory setting with the aid of an articulator.

The goal of the buildup is to restore parallelism of the occlusal table to Camper's plane and to the correct the VDO. It is important to design the

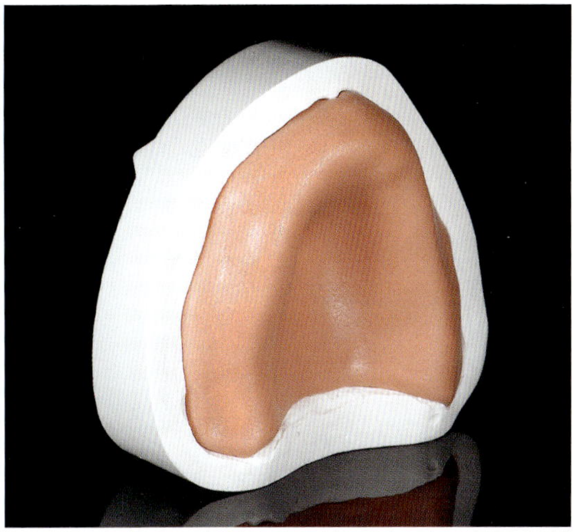

FIG 4-1 The contour and fit of the record base should already be as close as possible to the final denture base.

occlusal surfaces in a monoplane fashion, without any intercuspation. This allows the condyles to return to their physiologic centric position without any sagittal obstacles. The length of such preprosthetic measures depends on the severity, age, and adaptability of the patient and is to be determined and monitored by the skilled clinician.

Basic Recording Devices

Recording devices serve to register the physiologic centric relation as well as the VDO. In addition, they determine the esthetic and occlusal planes, which should be transversally parallel to the bipupillary line and sagittally parallel to Camper's plane.

Further, the contours and markings of the recording devices are invaluable communication tools and create a control template for the technician to follow with the subsequent setup.

The foundation of any recording device is a stable and torsion-free record base. As mentioned in previous chapters, vacuum-formed or light-cured baseplates come with several disadvantages. The use of a copolymer-based acrylic such as C-Plast (Candulor) is therefore a sensible option due to its dimensional stability. The contour and fitting of the record base should already be as close as possible to the final denture base (Fig 4-1).

The record bases are fabricated on the final master models. The fit as well as border length and thickness are determined by the valve margins previously established by the myofunctional impression and therefore correspond to the final denture base. Any undercut areas are to be blocked out with wax to avoid abrasion or fracturing of the master model.

The models are then soaked in lukewarm water for approximately 15 minutes, before an alginate-based separating agent is applied. The baseplate material is then prepared and adapted in a similar fashion to the fabrication of the custom impression tray, as outlined in chapter 2.

To construct the wax rims, a hard wax with a higher melting point should be selected. A softer wax can easily deform in the oral cavity during adjustments and the final recording procedure. Folded baseplate wax or preformed wax rims are both suitable options.

The width of the wax rims should not exceed a thickness of 8 mm in the posterior region and 4 mm in the anterior region. This avoids displacement of the tongue orally and enables the clinician to perform basic phonetic checks. The course of the rims is determined by a preliminary model analysis and should correspond as closely as possible to the future position of the prosthetic teeth.

The anterior height of the standardized wax rims to be built atop the record bases follows established median values: 20 to 22 mm in the maxilla and 16 to 18 mm in the mandible, for a total intervestibular distance of 36 to 40 mm. The reference point in the anterior vestibular fold lies approximately 10 mm lateral to the labial frenulum. A flexible ruler or an aid such as the OMP (Kolbeck Dental) is used to mark the desired height onto the anterior portion of the wax rim.

A heated rim former is used to reduce the initially overcontoured height of the wax rims. In the maxilla, the 6-mm-high posterior ledge of the rim former is placed into the hamular notches and rotated forward to melt the wax rims to the previously made anterior marking (Fig 4-2).

The principle is similar in the mandible; here, the posterior ledge of the wax rim points upward and is placed at the upper third of the retromolar pads and again rotated forward to reduce the wax rim to the anterior marking (Fig 4-3).

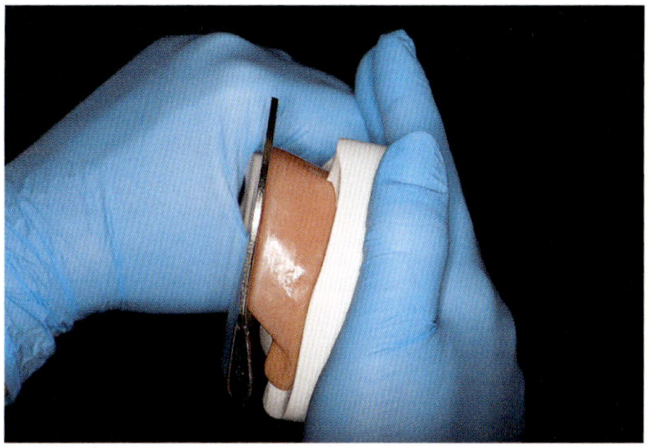

FIG 4-2 With the posterior ledge of the rim former positioned on the hamular notches, the wax rim is melted to the desired height.

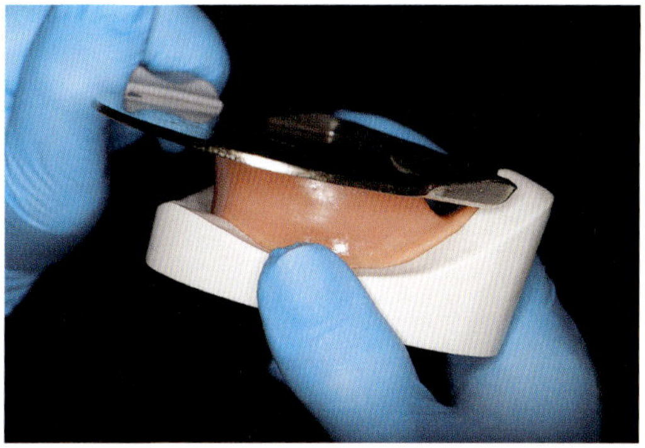

FIG 4-3 In the mandible, the rim former is rotated and the posterior ledge rests at the upper third of the retromolar pads.

Determination of the Individual Occlusal Height

As mentioned previously, centric relation varies depending on VDO. Thus, the correct occlusal height must be determined prior to the centric relation record.

For this purpose, the mandibular record base and wax rim are inserted into the patient's mouth and assessed. The occlusal plane can be determined by correcting the height and level of the wax rim to the equator of the relaxed tongue and anteriorly to the level of the upper edge of the relaxed lower lip. An additional reference is the middle or upper third of the retromolar pads. Here, too, the rim former is an ideal tool for the clinician to adjust the wax rim height and maintain parallelism of the occlusal plane (Fig 4-4a).

Next, the maxillary wax rim is inserted and assessed (Fig 4-4b). It must be adjusted in height until the freeway space is no less than 2 to 3 mm when the patient is instructed to count from 70 to 80. After confirmation of the freeway space, a Fox plane bite fork is used to check that the wax rims lie parallel to the interpupillary line and Camper's plane (Fig 4-5). Finally, the maxillary incisal edge position along with lip support and phonetics are assessed.

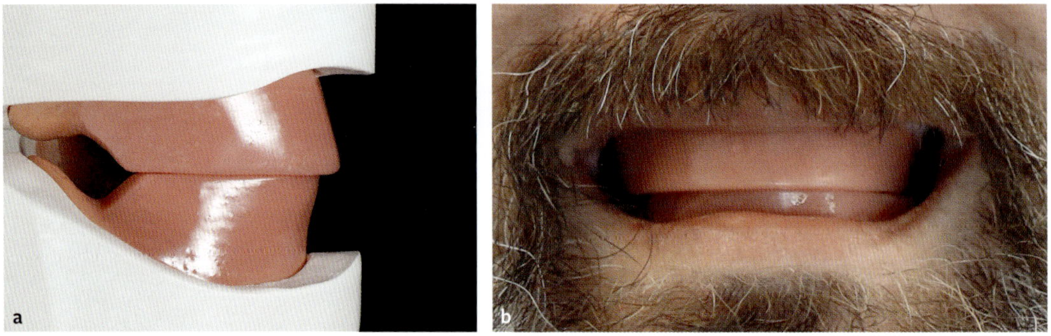

FIG 4-4 (*a*) The prepared wax rims must be strictly parallel to one another. The contours should already correspond with the approximate tooth positions based on landmarks. Especially in the mandible, a concave design allows room for the orbicularis oris muscles. (*b*) The wax rims are adjusted to the correct individual VDO.

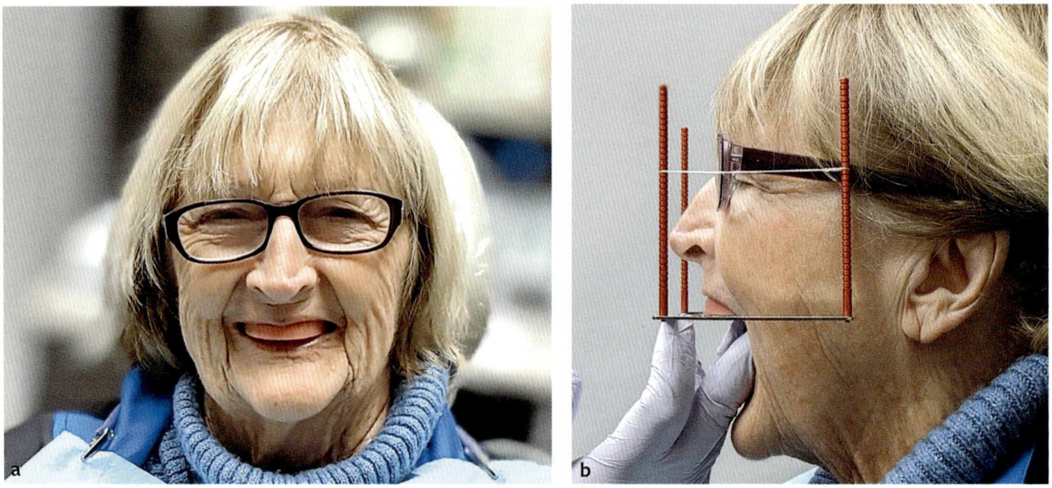

FIG 4-5 (*a*) The anterior plane typically runs parallel to the interpupillary line. (*b*) The occlusal plane of the maxillary wax rim is assessed with a Fox plane. It must run parallel to Camper's plane.

Recording Patient-Specific Data

It is essential to understand that the contours and markings of the wax rim create a control template, which the technician follows both for the articulation of the master models (median value articulation) as well as the subsequent tooth setup (Fig 4-6). As a minimum, the following data must be recorded to facilitate a predictable wax try-in appointment:

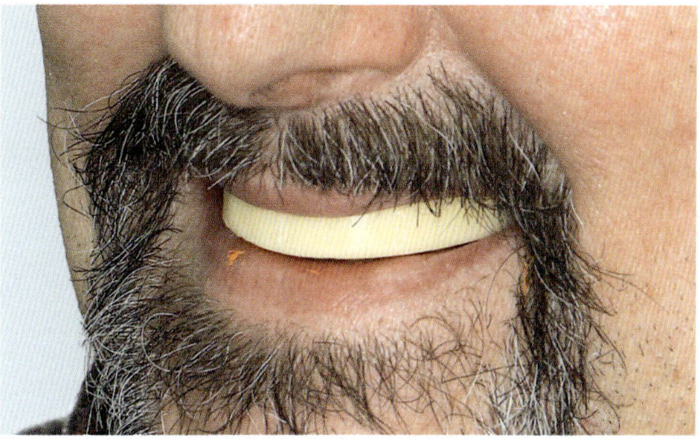

FIG 4-6 The maxillary wax rim has been contoured and marked. It contains all necessary information for the anterior composition of the prosthetic teeth.

- Incisal edge position of the central incisors for esthetics and phonetics
- Facial midline (the labial frenulum is not a reliable landmark)
- Ala lines as a reference for anterior width and canine positions
- High smile line of the upper lip to determine reveal
- Contour of the lower lip when smiling to determine the curve of the anterior composition
- Lip and cheek support

Customized Wax Rims

To reduce time-consuming adjustments of the wax rims prior to determining centric relation, the clinician is encouraged to provide the laboratory technician with a preliminary bite record and patient-specific data for the length of the maxillary wax rim during the previous appointment.

The Papillameter is used to measure the length of the relaxed upper lip relative to the incisal papilla (Fig 4-7). This measurement should be repeated two to three times, ideally with the patient standing upright. Frush developed norm guidelines that take the age and gender of the patient into account (Table 4-1).

TABLE 4-1 Frush's norms for upper lip–incisive papilla distance according to age and gender

Age	~28 years	~40 years	~50 years	~65 years	~70+ years
Male	+1.5 to +2.5 mm	+1.0 to +2.0 mm	+0.5 to +1.0 mm	–1.0 to 0.0 mm	–2.0 to –4.0 mm
Female	+2.0 to +3.0 mm	+1.5 to +2.0 mm	+1.0 to +2.0 mm	+0.5 to +1.0 mm	0.0 to –1.0 mm

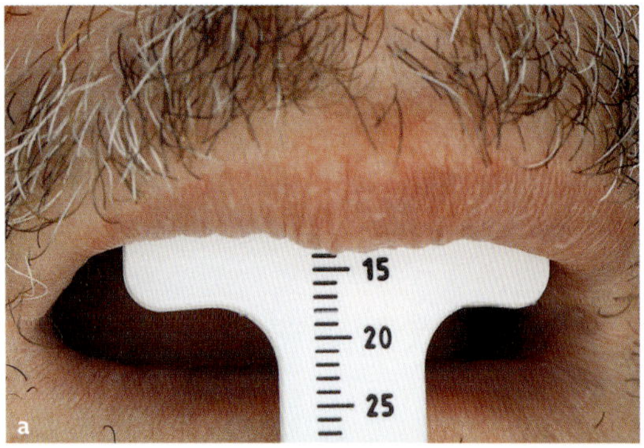

FIG 4-7 (*a*) The Papillameter measures the length of the relaxed upper lip relative to the incisal papilla. (*b*) The individual values of the Papillameter are recorded with a sliding caliper on the master cast. (*c*) The height of the wax rim now corresponds to the individual value.

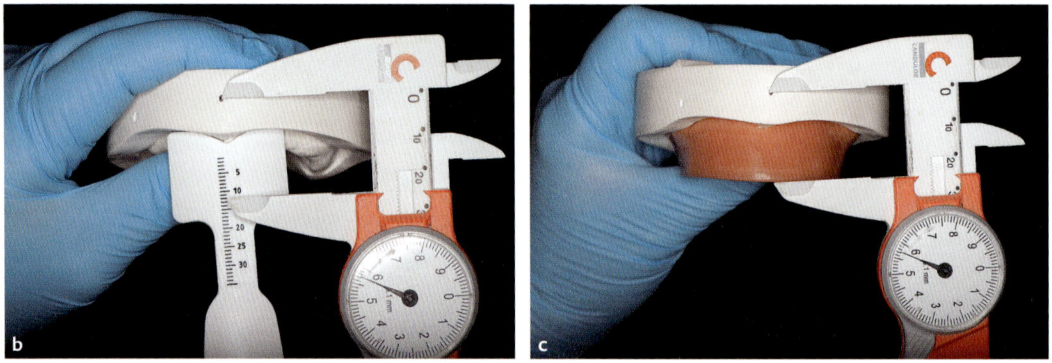

A preliminary record of centric relation and VDO further reduces the time spent on adjusting the wax rims. A simple-to-use instrument for this purpose is the Centric Tray (Ivoclar). The preliminary VDO can be determined as follows:

1. The clinician applies two dots on the patient's chin and tip of the nose with a skin-friendly marker.
2. The patient is instructed to hum the letter "M" continuously.
3. The distance between the two arbitrary dots measured with a sliding caliper represents the vertical dimension of rest, or VDR (Fig 4-8).
4. The distance of VDR is reduced by 2 to 3 mm to take freeway space into account, and the caliper is set accordingly. This represents a *preliminary* VDO.
5. The Centric Tray is loaded with a silicone putty and inserted into the mouth (Fig 4-9).

FIG 4-8 While the patient continuously hums the letter "M," the distance between two arbitrary marks on the nose and chin is measured. This distance corresponds with the resting position.

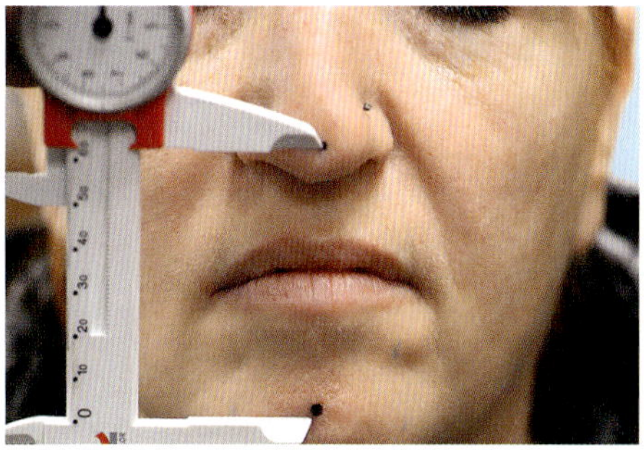

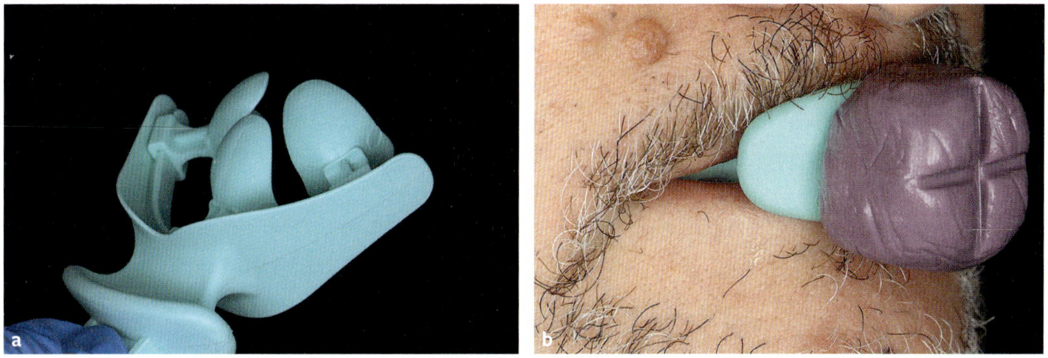

FIG 4-9 (*a*) The Centric Tray is an easy-to-use instrument to record preliminary centric relation and VDO. (*b*) The Centric Tray in situ without the use of a facebow.

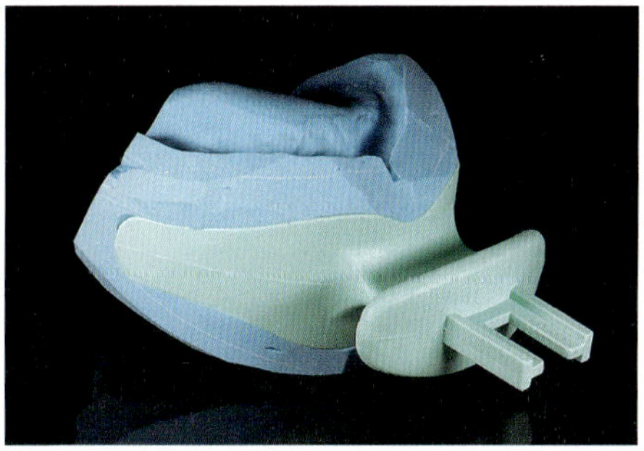

FIG 4-10 Preliminary record of centric relation and VDO.

6. The patient is instructed the slowly close into the soft putty. Simultaneously, the clinician uses the caliper and the arbitrary dots to control the closing movement until the predetermined VDO is reached.
7. The patient is then instructed to stop the closing movement.
8. Once the putty has set, the Centric Tray is removed (Fig 4-10).

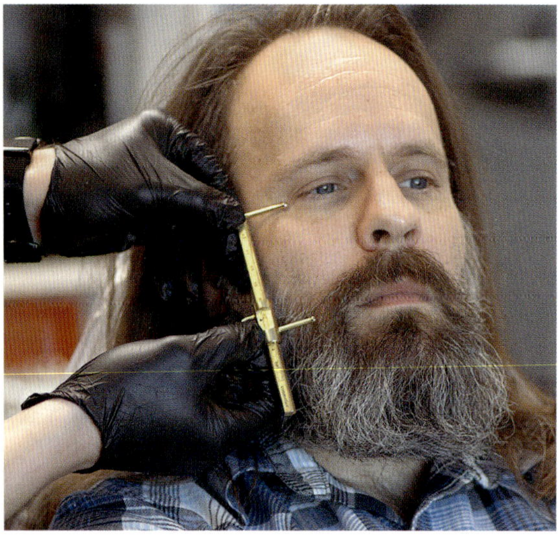

FIG 4-11 The distance between the corner of the eye and the corner of the mouth is similar to the distance between the anterior nasal spine and the lower edge of the chin.

An alternative option to determine preliminary VDO is with the use of a Verti-Corder. Here the preliminary VDO is determined by comparing the distance between the corner of the eye and the corner of the mouth with the distance between the anterior nasal spine and the lower edge of the chin (Fig 4-11).

Existing sets of dentures that are either correct in VDO or have been corrected during the preprosthetic treatment may also be used as an aid to determine preliminary VDO.

The measurements from the Papillameter and the preliminary record enable the laboratory technician to articulate the master models and fabricate patient-specific wax rims (Figs 4-12 to 4-14). An additional advantage of the Centric Tray is its ability to be connected to the UTS 3D facebow (Ivoclar). By using a facebow at this stage, the maxillary master model is already correctly oriented spatially in the articulator.

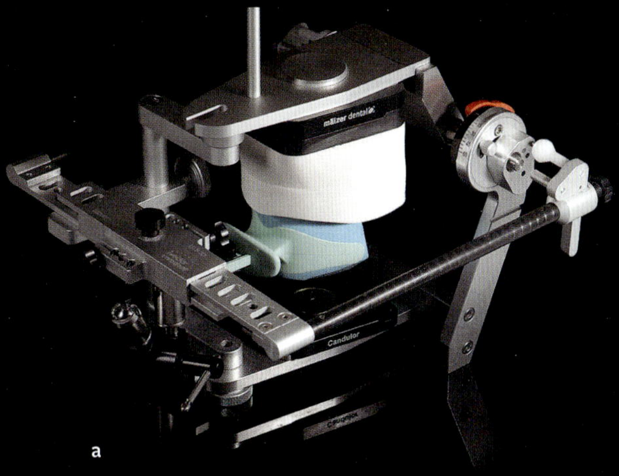

a

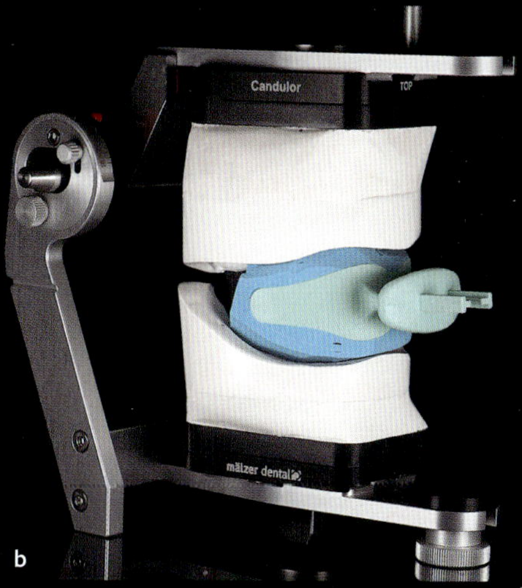

b

FIG 4-12 (*a*) Maxillary master model articulated with the preliminary record and the UTS 3D facebow. (*b*) Completed preliminary articulation of the master models.

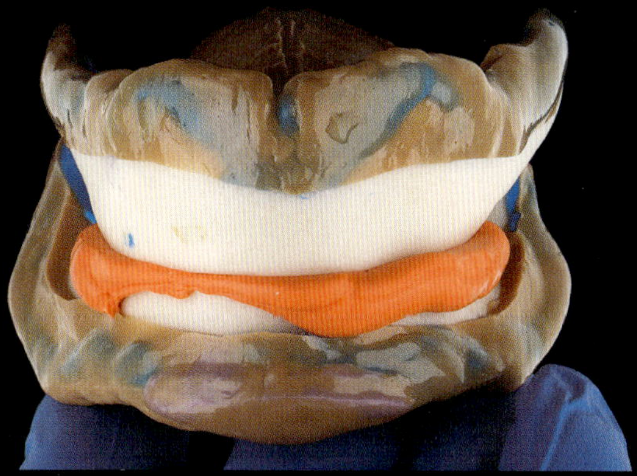

FIG 4-13 As an alternative, a preliminary record of centric relation and VDO may be obtained with the myofunctional impression trays.

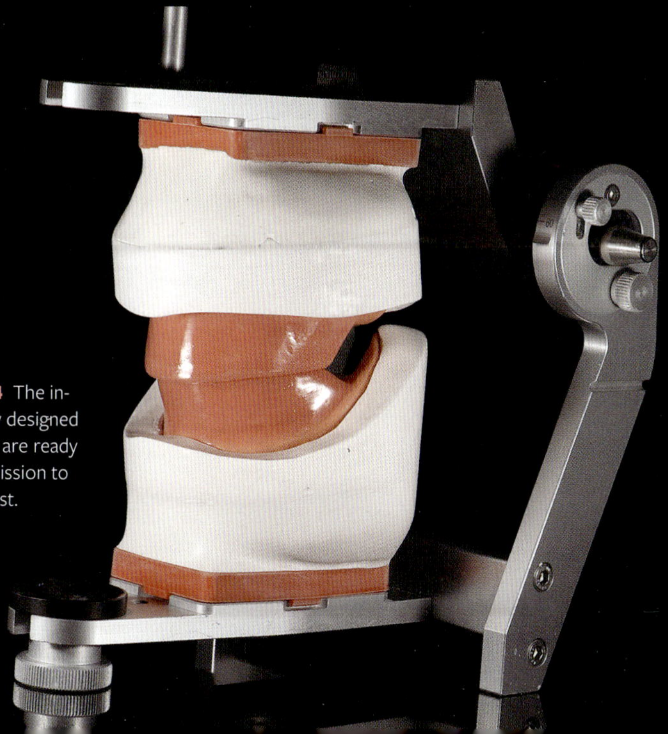

FIG 4-14 The individually designed wax rims are ready for submission to the dentist.

Maxillomandibular Record with Wax Rims

Once the final VDO is determined, the wax rims are contoured and marked as described above, the occlusal and esthetic planes are verified with the Fox plane, and the final record of centric relation can commence.

The patient must be able to close to the final bite height without interference. The clinician will create notches in the posterior occlusal surfaces of the wax rims, which will be used for indexing the registration material. Vertical lines in the areas of the canines and second premolars in both arches are carved. The patient is then instructed to open and close several times, alternating with laterotrusive movements. The clinician will observe if the vertical lines are congruent each time. If this is the case, the position is registered bilaterally with a rigid bite registration material.

Note: Recording centric relation with conventional wax rims is not recommended in most cases. The risk of recording pathologic or habitual intercuspation positions is relatively high, which frequently means physiologic centric relation is not captured. The technique should only be applied if an instrument-aided registration (as described later in the section titled "Maxillomandibular Record According to Gerber/McGrain") is not indicated.

Protrusive Record

After VDO and centric relation records are created, the silicone key is removed, disinfected, and placed into a labeled bag. With the wax rim templates still in situ, the patient is instructed to move the mandible into a maximum protrusive position. Due to Christensen's phenomenon, the wax rims will disocclude posteriorly. While remaining in this position, the clinician injects registration material bilaterally into the gaps. The technician will use this protrusive record to program the condylar elements of the articulator, which will later aid in the creation of the individually equilibrated, polyvalent occlusal geometry during the laboratory remount. **The protrusive record must be placed in a separate bag after disinfection and labeled accordingly.**

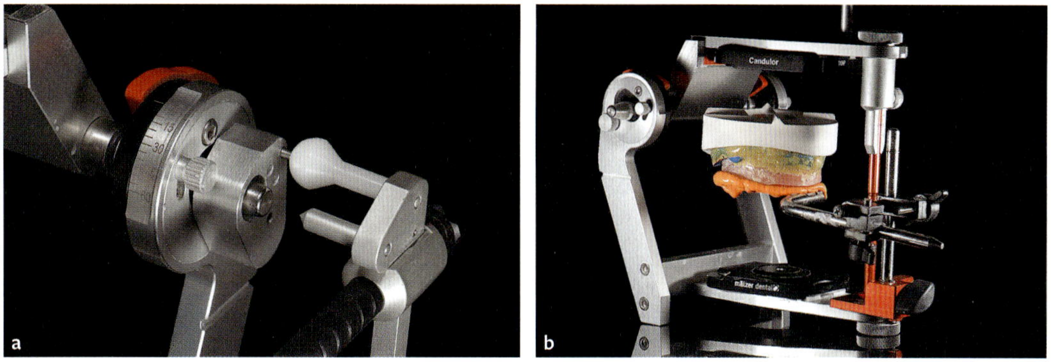

FIG 4-15 (*a*) Universal adapters are available for some articulator systems to accommodate different makes of facebows. It is important that both the clinician and technician are knowledgeable about the different systems. (*b*) Transfer of a Denar face-bow record to a CA 3.0 L articulator with a transfer jig.

Facebow Record

A facebow record is a crucial tool in the denture fabrication process that is used to capture the relationship between the patient's maxilla (or, in the case of the kinetic facebow, the patient's mandible) and the TMJs. One of the primary benefits of using a facebow record is its ability to provide a spatially correct representation of the patient's jaw positioning as well as esthetic parameters. This information is invaluable in planning and executing prosthetic treatment.

By accurately capturing the spatial relationship between the patient's jaws and TMJs, a facebow record helps to ensure proper dynamic occlusion. This is necessary to achieve functional and esthetic outcomes in dentures and other forms of full-mouth rehabilitation. When providing these restorative treatments, it is crucial to replicate the patient's unique jaw positioning to ensure positional stability and proper masticatory function. A facebow record provides the necessary data to accurately articulate the master models and guide the fabrication process.

Additionally, a facebow record enables improved communication between dental professionals. By documenting the precise relationship between the patient's jaws and TMJ hinge axis, clinicians and laboratory technicians can share valuable information and collaborate effectively on treatment plans (Fig 4-15).

If the maxillary master model has not already been mounted with a facebow via a Centric Tray, the record is now created by using a bite fork attached to the joint assembly of the adjusted transfer bow.

Maxillomandibular Record According to Gerber/McGrain

Compared to manual registration, the use of a central bearing device can yield far more accurate and reproducible results. Authors like Bosshart state an accuracy rate of 95%. In case of a faulty record, the additional time and cost of rearticulation and reset of the denture teeth can be frustrating to the clinician, the patient, and the laboratory technician. It therefore seems expedient to use a method that typically avoids such risks.

The intraoral tracing, sometimes called the *Gothic arch tracing*, is particularly indicated in cases where a reproducible manual record cannot be expected or obtained. The following paragraphs describe the fabrication of such a device in the clinical setting.

After the wax rims have been adjusted as described in the previous paragraphs, the so-called "striking plate" of a central bearing device, such as the CRS-10 (Candulor), is heated over a Bunsen burner and melted 1-mm deep into the mandibular wax rim. It is important to maintain both the established occlusal plane and the height of the wax rim. The correct size of the maxillary pin support holder is then melted about 3 to 5 mm deep into the maxillary wax rim. The scribing pin is screwed into the thread and adjusted to the height of the wax rim (Fig 4-16). This way, the previously established VDO is preserved. **The screw should be secured with a drop of sticky wax or compound.**

Once cooled, the maxillary wax rim is reduced to the level of the pin support plate. By doing so, any interference between the templates is eliminated and only the scribing pin and the striking plate will contact in situ.

Note: If the clinician has provided preliminary records as described previously in this chapter, the intraoral tracer assembly can also be constructed in an articulator by the laboratory technician ahead of the record appointment (Fig 4-17). The laboratory provides the clinician with a customized maxillary wax rim for contouring and all relevant markings, along with the mandibular wax rim containing the striking plate and the scribing pin on a separate maxillary record base. This approach saves valuable chair time and adds an additional level of accuracy.

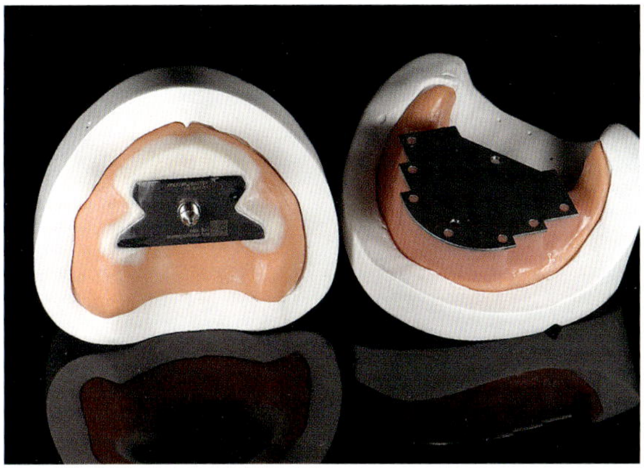

FIG 4-16 The intraoral tracer assembly ready for final records.

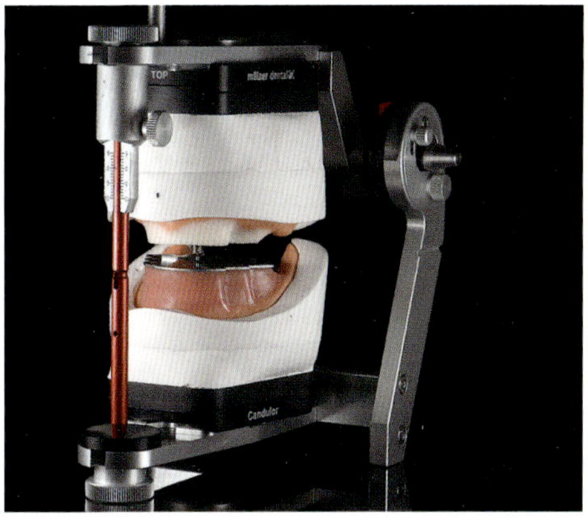

FIG 4-17 Intraoral tracer constructed beforehand in the laboratory. This workflow saves valuable chair time and adds an additional level of accuracy.

The prepared registration device is now inserted into the patient's mouth. Once more, the VDO is confirmed and corrected via the scribing pin, if necessary. No interference between the templates must occur, and the scribing pin and striking plate must be clearly visible to the clinician.

It is recommended to explain the procedure to the patient beforehand and allow the patient to practice performing excursive movements with the registration device prior to the actual recording.

To begin the recording procedure, the striking plate is colored with a nontoxic wax crayon or similar instrument. The patient is asked to move the mandible to the left and back to the center, followed by a movement to the right and back to the center again. Then the patient is instructed to perform a protrusive movement. The use of hand signals can help the patient perform the excursions in the desired order.

In most cases, an arrowhead or "Gothic arch" becomes visible on the striking plate (Fig 4-18). The tip of the arrowhead, or the zenith point, represents physiologic centric relation. As an added safety measure, the mandibular template is removed, and a crosshair symbol is drawn over the zenith point. The remainder

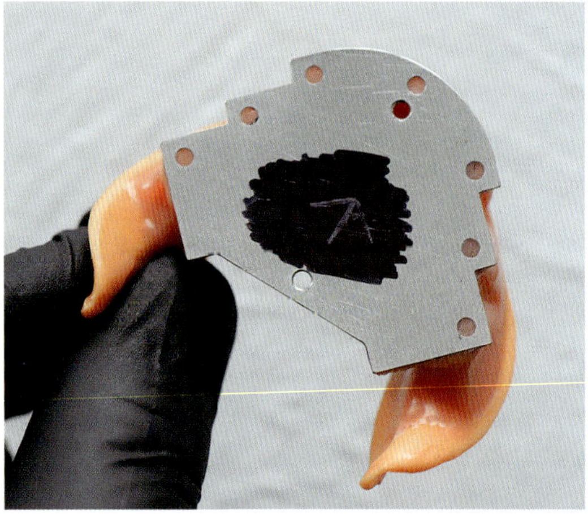

FIG 4-18 Classic "arrowhead" pattern. The apex of the tracing indicates physiologic centric relation.

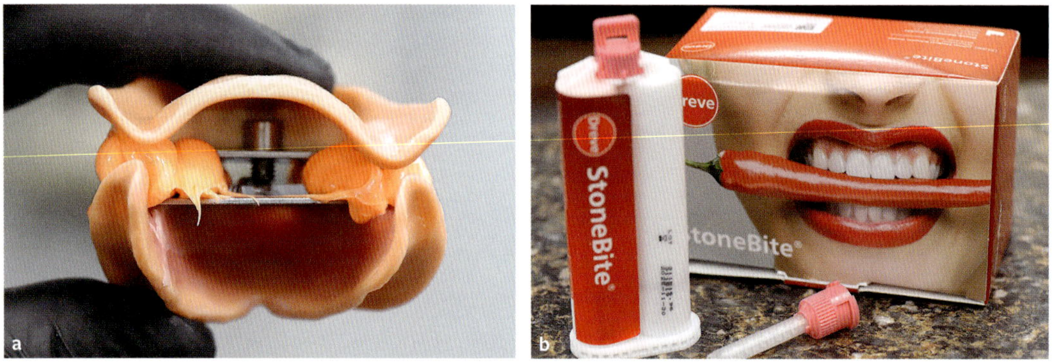

FIG 4-19 (*a*) The intraoral tracing is completed and keyed with rigid bite registration material. (*b*) A rigid registration material like StoneBite (Dreve) is preferable over more flexible options.

of the tracing pattern is colored with wax crayon again. Then the procedure is repeated. If the tip of the arrow is congruent with the first tracing, the beveled hole of the plastic tile included in the tracer kit is placed over the zenith point and, depending on the system, secured with a screw or compound.

The mandibular template is reinserted, and the patient is asked to open and close several times. If the scribing pin snaps effortlessly into the beveled hole, physiologic centric relation is confirmed and bilaterally keyed with a rigid registration material (Fig 4-19).

If the patient's excursive movements appear tense or inhibited, it can be beneficial to instruct the patient to remain in the determined relation for a few minutes prior to registration. If no tension or discomfort is reported or observed, the registration is indexed. Otherwise, the reason for the inhibition must be diagnosed and clarified. Additional preprosthetic treatment may be indicated.

Combined Maxillomandibular Record with Kinetic Facebow Record

The maxillomandibular record with an intraoral tracing as described above may also be combined with a kinetic facebow record. The Gerber Facebow (Condylator) is a sophisticated instrument used to trace the sagittal condylar slope and to transfer the relation between the patient's occlusal plane and the condylar hinge axis to an adjustable articulator.

The mensuration of the sagittal condylar joint path is carried out *after* the determination of VDO and *before* the final recording of centric relation. The scribing plate of the Gerber-Transfer-Registration Set-106 (Condylator) features two forward-pointing guide pins onto which the facebow is attached (Fig 4-20).

The clinician determines the external condyle poles either via palpation or arbitrarily via a line from each tragus to the ala of the nose. The reference point typically lies on this line 13 mm anterior to the tragus and is marked with a skin-friendly pen (Fig 4-21).

The left and right arms of the Gerber facebow must be in an upright position to avoid any injury to the patient! The facebow is then attached to the guide pins of the scribing plate, and the lateral arms of the facebow are equipped with the pencil assemblies. The arms are adjusted so that the indicator rods or the pencil leads are aligned with the markings of the external condyle poles (Fig 4-22). Once in place, the positions are fixed with the screws on each side of the lateral arms.

To record the sagittal condyle path, the registration card included with the kit is held with one hand against the patient's temple. The millimeter grid is aligned with the lateral orientation rods of the facebow. **Note:** The orientation rods must be parallel to the occlusal plane (ie, Camper's plane; Fig 4-23).

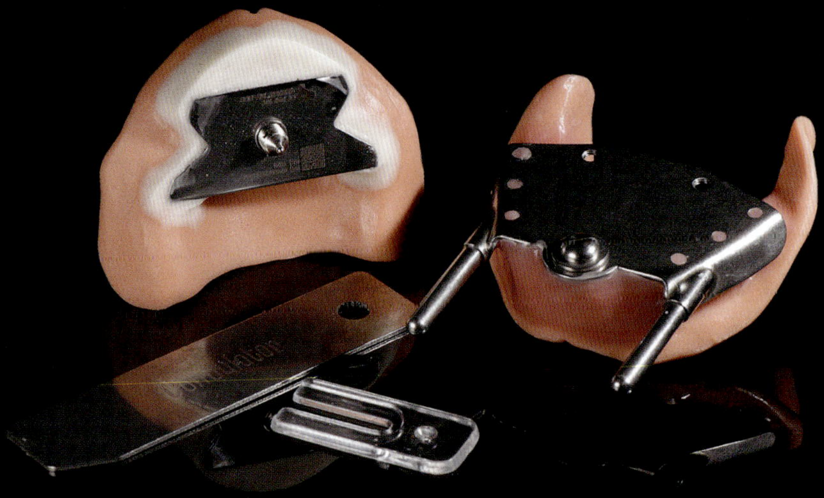

FIG 4-20 The Gerber-Transfer-Registration Set-106 features two forward-pointing guide pins onto which the facebow is attached.

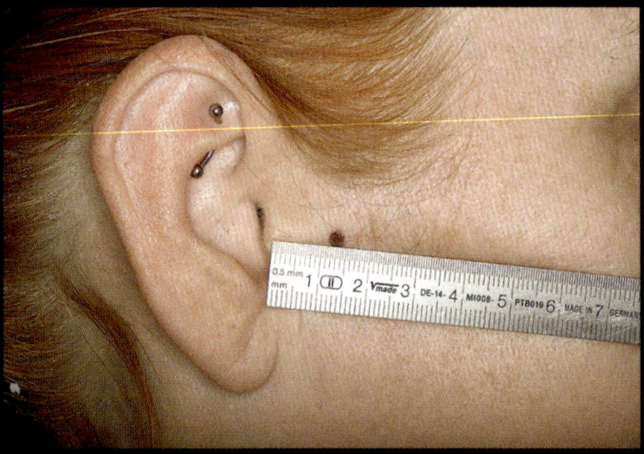

FIG 4-21 The reference point typically lies on this line 13 mm anterior to the tragus and is marked with a skin-friendly pen.

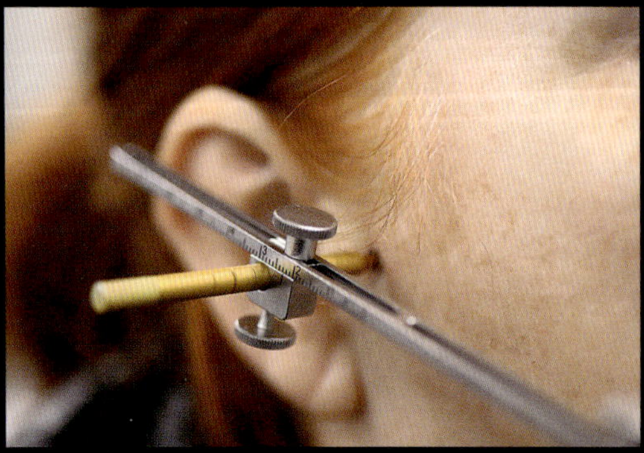

FIG 4-22 The indicator rods are aligned with the markings of the external condyle poles.

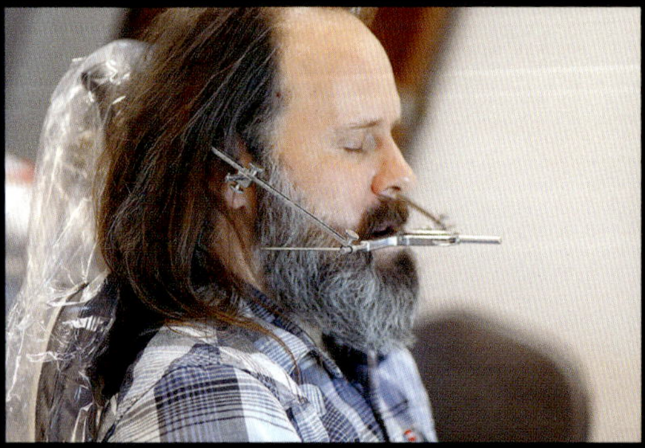

FIG 4-23 The lateral reference rod is parallel to Camper's plane.

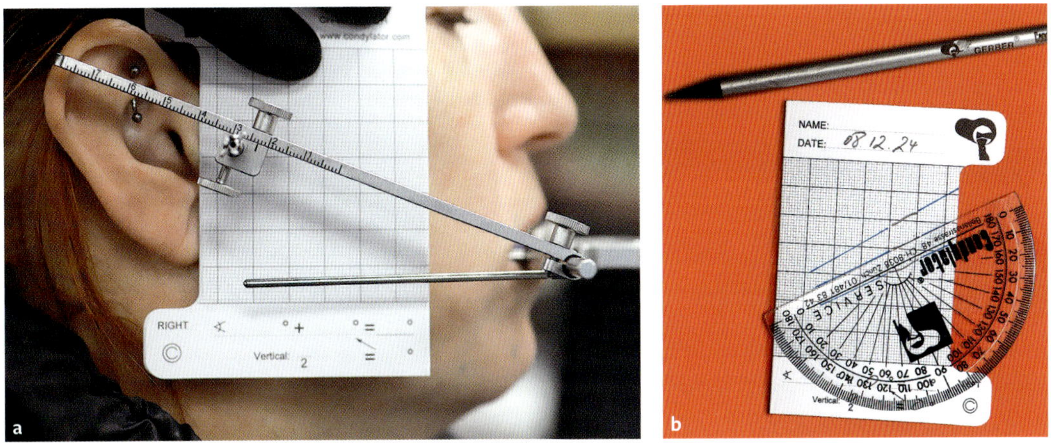

FIG 4-24 (*a*) The horizontal lines of the grid on the registration card must be aligned with the reference rod of the Gerber facebow. (*b*) Evaluation of the condylography with a protractor.

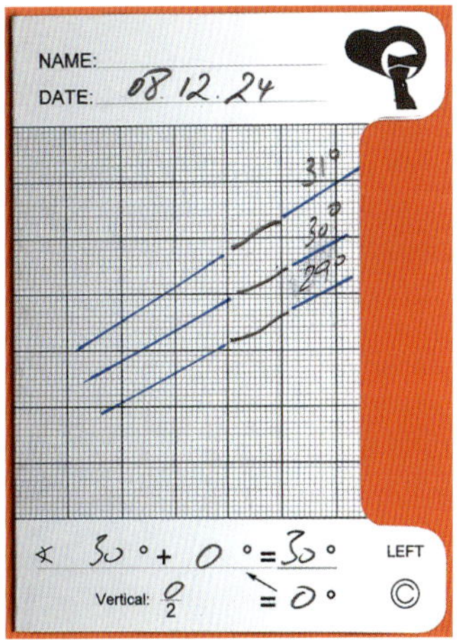

FIG 4-25 The average value of three joint path measurements determines the sagittal condyle angle. If the tracing was conducted with an opened VDO, half a degree must be added for each millimeter.

Measurements are conducted separately on each side. The graphite pen is extended from its cartridge and must be in solid contact with the registration card. The patient is instructed to perform a protrusive movement while the intraoral scribing pin and the striking plate remain in contact. The graphite pen will trace the sagittal condyle path onto the registration card (Fig 4-24).

At the end of the protrusive movement, the graphite pen is retracted, and the patient is asked to return to centric relation. It is recommended to repeat the procedure three times, with the card being moved upward or downward for each tracing (Fig 4-25). The procedure is then repeated on the other side.

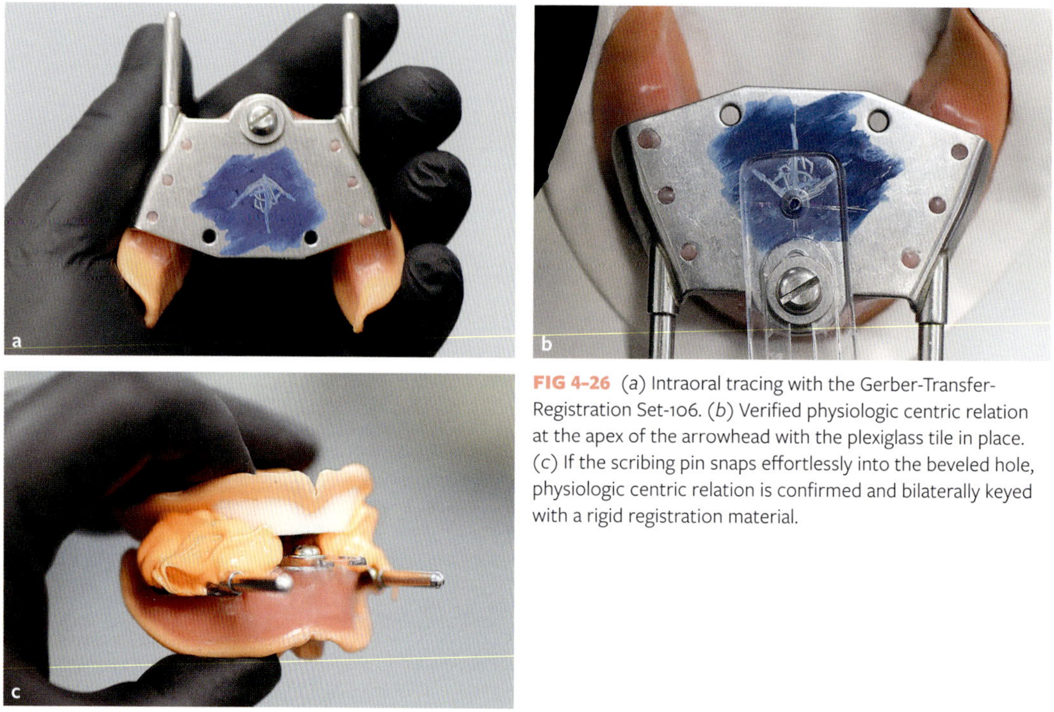

FIG 4-26 (*a*) Intraoral tracing with the Gerber-Transfer-Registration Set-106. (*b*) Verified physiologic centric relation at the apex of the arrowhead with the plexiglass tile in place. (*c*) If the scribing pin snaps effortlessly into the beveled hole, physiologic centric relation is confirmed and bilaterally keyed with a rigid registration material.

Finally, the facebow is carefully removed from the patient. **It is critical that the adjusted facebow is not altered in any way before the master models are mounted!**

The intraoral tracer assembly remains in the patient's mouth, and the final record of the maxillomandibular relationship is completed as described in the previous section (Fig 4-26).

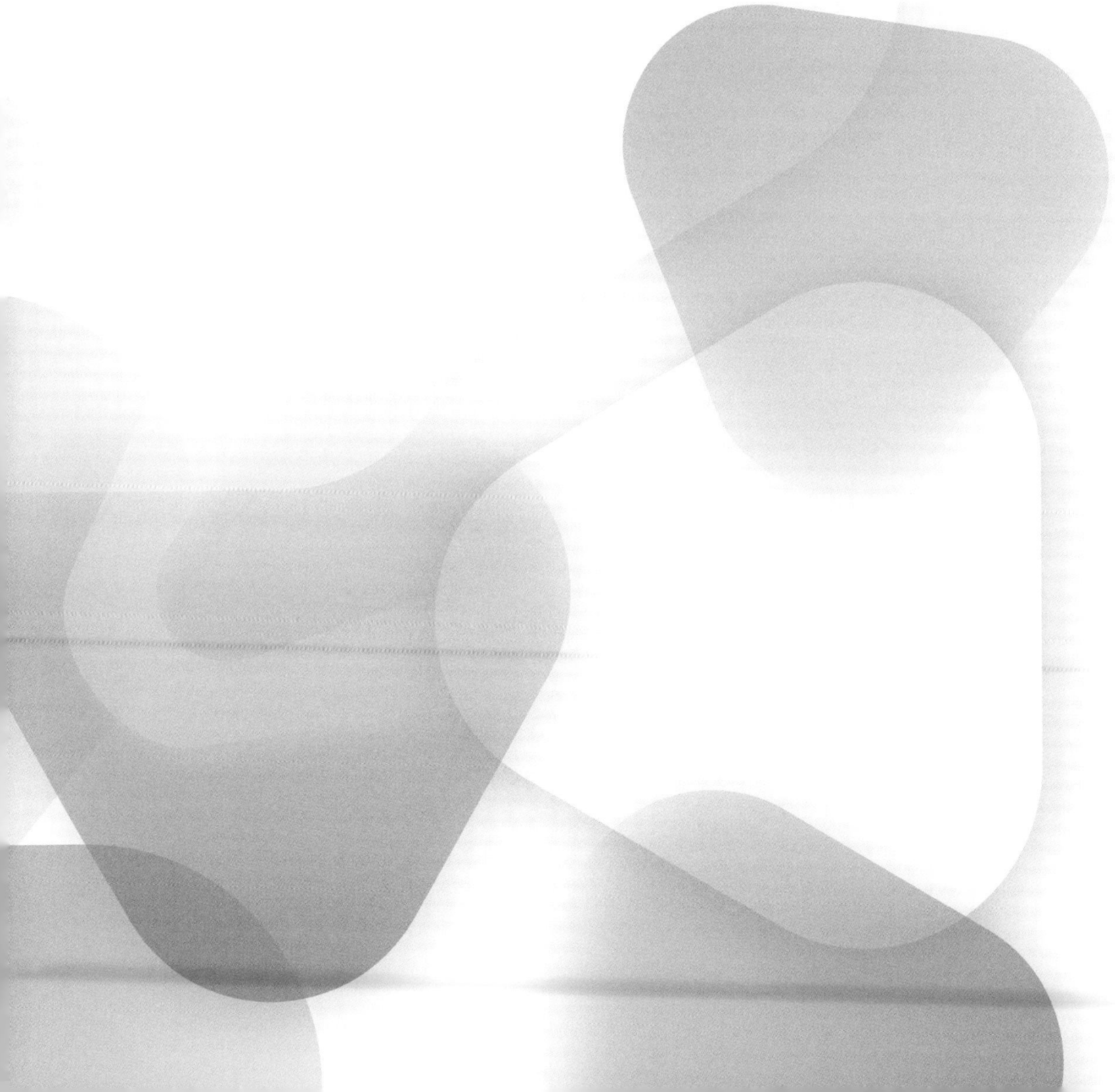

5

MODEL ASSEMBLY

Average-Value Assembly

The advantages of using a facebow record for model assembly have been discussed in chapter 4. In the absence of such a record, the master casts are mounted following average values.

Most articulator systems are designed with the upper and lower members of the instrument parallel to Camper's plane. Therefore, the mandibular wax rim may be aligned with the aid of a rubber band and the symphysis pointer inserted into the incisal pin. With the help of modeling clay, the mandibular model is now positioned along Camper's plane and within the Bonwill triangle. The centric relation record is added, along with the maxillary master cast, and fixated. The maxillary model is then mounted with ISO Type 2 plaster or, ideally, with a low-expansion mounting stone.

Once the plaster has set and is trimmed, the modeling clay is removed and the articulator is turned upside down, and the mandibular cast is mounted.

The average-value articulation is a fundamental procedure and doesn't require much additional explanation.

Tip: Assembling the models and the centric relation record with two spent burs, nails, or wooden craft sticks and hot glue is a reliable and clean method that does not cause unsightly abrasion to the model bases. Rubber bands holding the models and registration together, however, are not recommended.

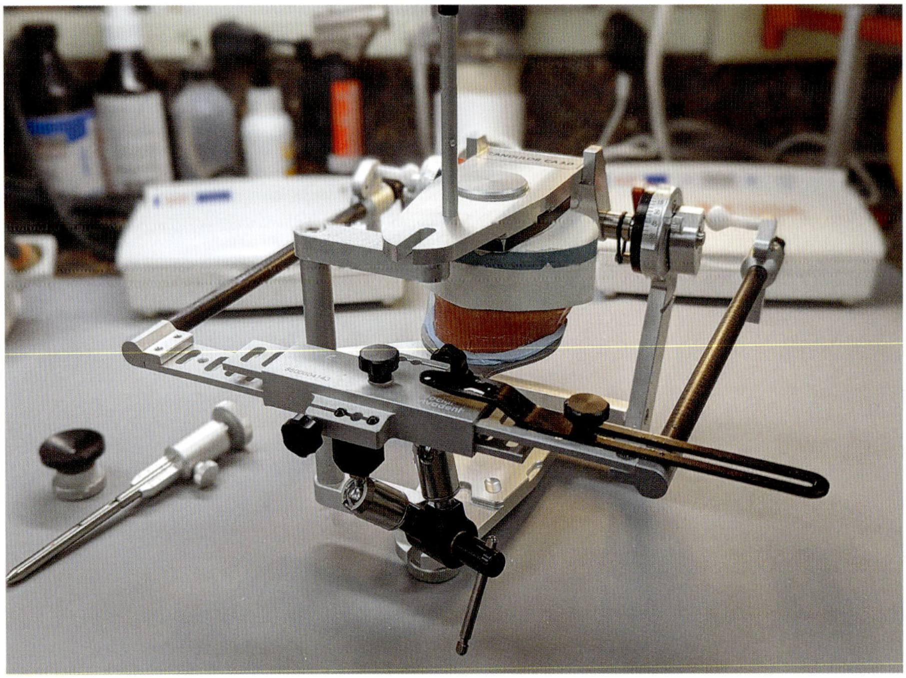

FIG 5-1 Ivoclar UTS 3D facebow.

Patient-Specific Assembly with Facebow Record

When using facebow records, both the clinician and technician must be familiar with the system used. Depending on the system, additional parts are necessary to transfer the record to the articulator. Figures 5-1 to 5-4 show some of the different systems used.

Typically, the maxillary cast is secured to the bite fork or transport jig and articulated first. The mandibular model is then fixated with the centric relation record and articulated subsequently.

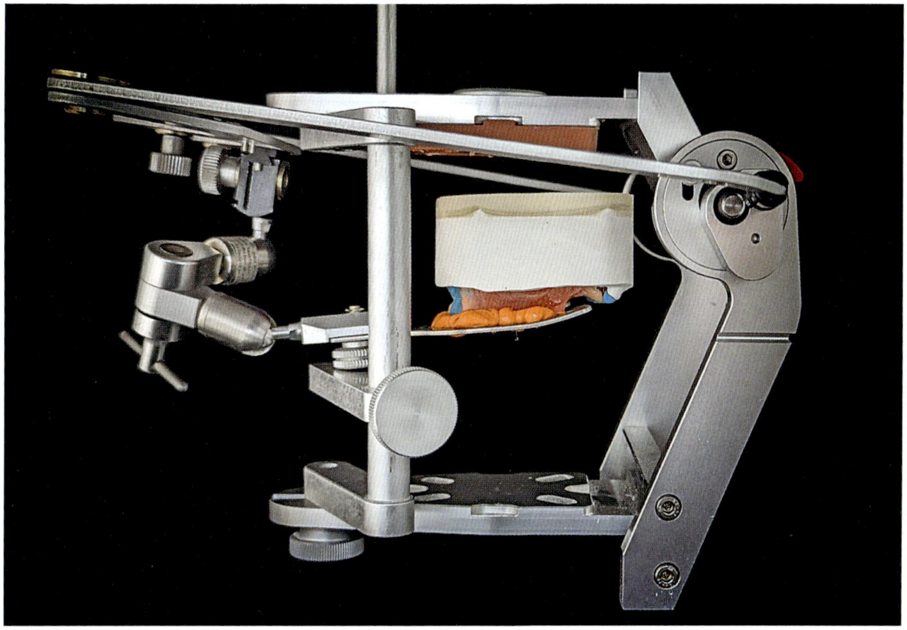

FIG 5-2 SAM facebow.

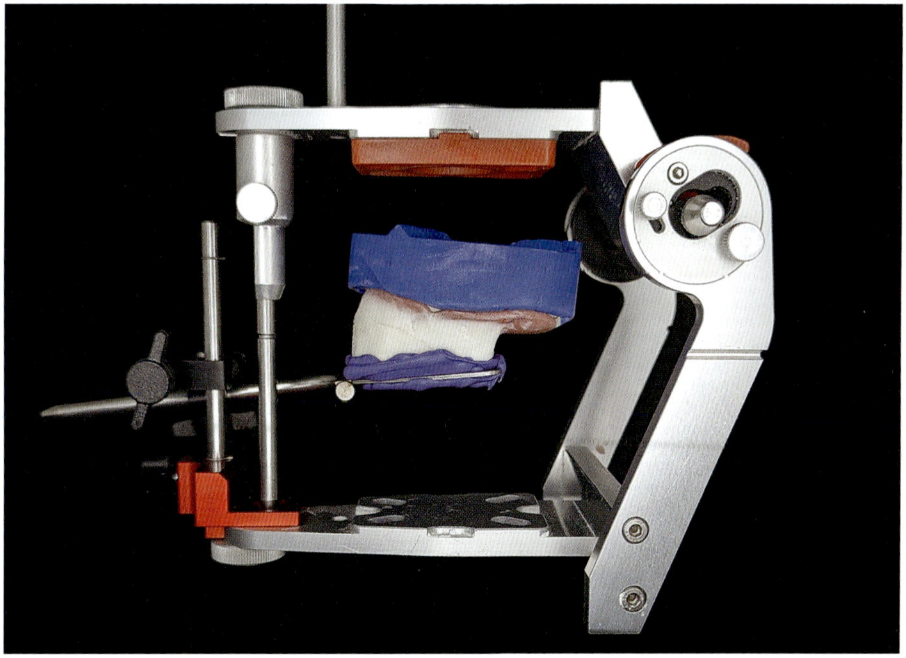

FIG 5-3 Denar facebow.

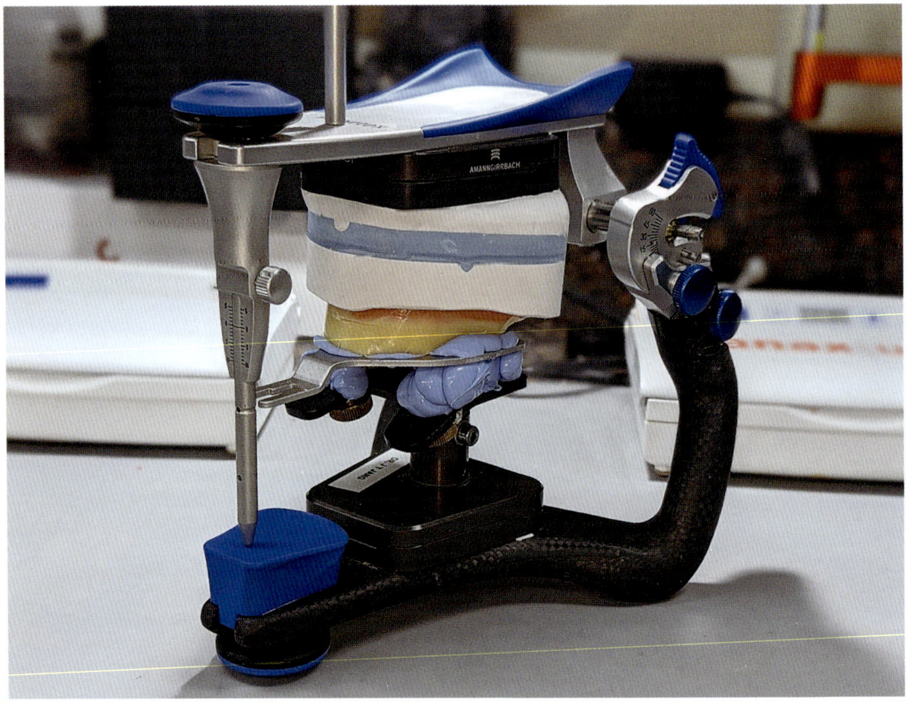

FIG 5-4 Artex facebow on transport jig.

Assembly with Kinetic Gerber Facebow in the Condylator

For assembly with the kinetic Gerber facebow, the facebow record is attached to the stand, and the graphite pens/guide rods are aligned with the centers of the Condylator joints (Fig 5-5). The height must only be adjusted via the frontal guide screw. The mandibular model is mounted first. Once the mounting stone has set, the facebow is removed. The registration is then used to articulate the maxillary model accordingly.

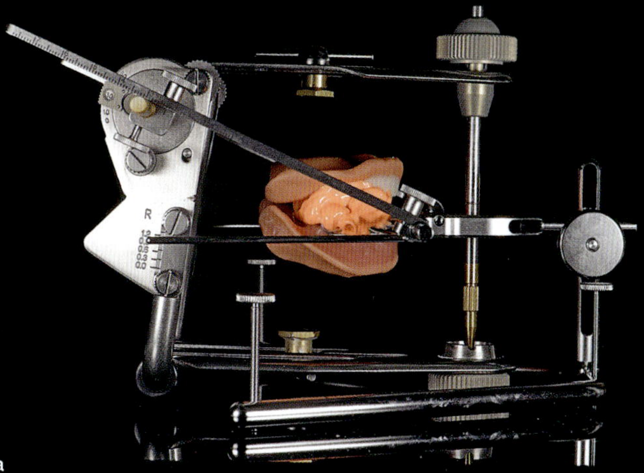

a

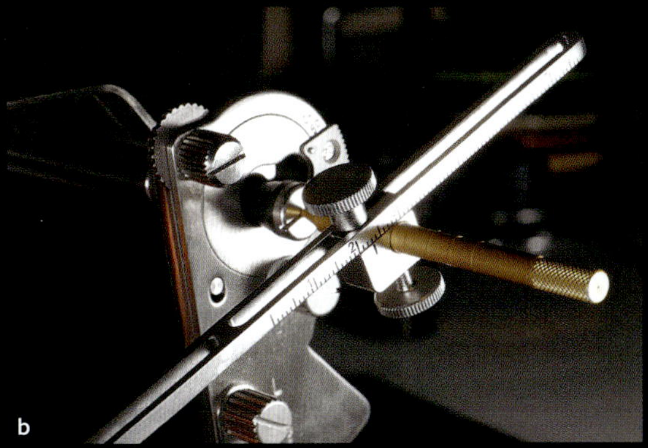

b

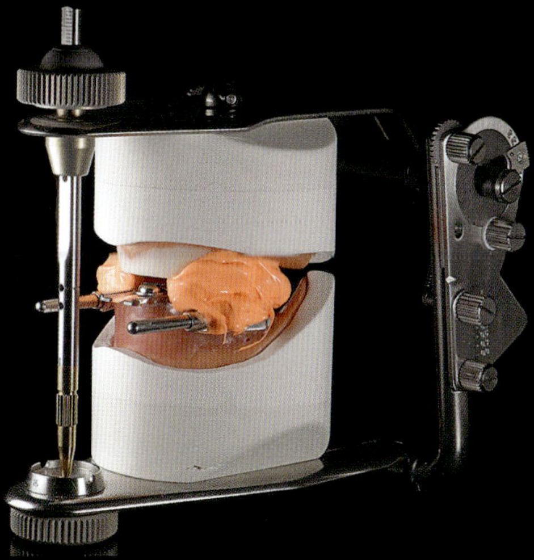

c

FIG 5-5 (*a*) Gerber facebow with Condylator. (*b*) The condyle pointer is precisely aligned with the articulator condylar axis. (*c*) Completed assembly of the Gerber facebow in the Condylator.

6

THE MODEL ANALYSIS

Purpose of the Model Analysis

One of the most important aspects of complete denture design is the correct setup of the artificial teeth. The static and dynamic contact relationships between the arches directly affect positional stability. While most traditional and contemporary experts agree on the importance of bilaterally balanced occlusion, the ridge-adequate setup of the posterior teeth is of equal, if not higher, importance. Human beings tend to chew predominantly on one side, during which the food bolus cancels occlusion until the very last phase of the masticatory cycle. Therefore, all pairs of antagonistic teeth must be stable under unilateral load, a concept that has been described by Gerber as "autonomous chewing stability." He defined the concept as follows:

- Each pair of opposing posterior teeth does not destabilize the denture under occlusal load.
- All masticatory forces are directed in their entirety perpendicular to the denture-bearing area.
- No occlusal contacts occur on inclined planes.

Masticatory forces are transferred via the occlusal surfaces toward the underlying alveolar ridges; where and at what angle determines chewing stability. Over a century ago, Gysi determined that these forces should be directed at an angle perpendicular to the crest of the ridge.

Forces acting on inclined planes are deflected as horizontal thrusts, leading to a forward gliding of the dentures, which can be highly destructive to the underlying anatomy and/or implants. Therefore, it is common knowledge to position the largest masticatory unit, usually the first molars, onto the lowest area of the mandibular ridge. This also applies to the maxilla; the first molars should be positioned onto the highest area of the posterior ridge.

Difficulties can arise if the highest and lowest areas diverge in the maxilla and mandible. Here, we must find a compromise and determine the most logical areas for the antagonistic pairs of first molars.

As previously stated, the masticatory forces are transferred via the occlusal surfaces to the ridges. If these forces act on a perpendicular surface, the dentures will be stable. However, the course of the residual ridge is rarely straight but rather sloped and inclined when compared to the occlusal plane. For this reason, we must aim to set the posterior teeth parallel to the ridge contours. In most cases, we can use the model analysis to find where the lowest/highest areas coincide, or we can determine common areas that are parallel to the occlusal plane and to each other.

In borderline cases, it may even be necessary to divert the prosthetic occlusal plane from the natural plane in order to achieve a ridge-adequate arrangement. This might appear unusual but is functionally appropriate.

The goal of the model analysis is therefore to identify where the posterior teeth may be positioned in relation to the residual ridge to avoid a dislocation of the dentures under function. The model analysis further determines what sequence of posterior teeth may be set up and which areas may not be exposed to masticatory forces.

Step-by-Step Basic Model Analysis

Several approaches to model analysis exist today based on the desired occlusal scheme and, logically, the selected tooth design for each individual case. These slightly different approaches all have merit and may include, for example, the addition of so-called "correction lines." These aim to create a triangular functional space extending buccal and lingual of the center of the ridge crest. This allows for the use of fully anatomical teeth with physiologic ABC contacts. The masticatory surface of this type of posterior tooth naturally is wider buccolingually, therefore requiring a wider stable zone.

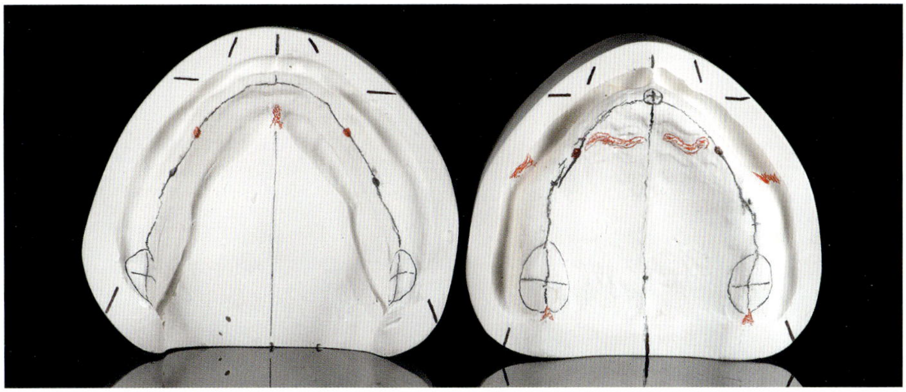

FIG 6-1 The metric midlines, estimates of the first premolar positions, the lowest/highest points of the residual ridges, and the basic static lines are marked.

Another variation pertains to the stop line, which determines the dorsal boundary where teeth may no longer be functionally loaded based on the ascension of the mandibular ridge contour. Gerber found that any masticatory forces on an inclined plane lead to a protraction or forward gliding of either or both dentures. He therefore determined the stop line to be placed strictly at the beginning of the ascending ramus.

This type of stop line inevitably leads to a shortened row of posterior teeth in most cases. Lerch therefore introduced a compromise in which teeth may still be loaded on an inclined plane of up to 22.5 degrees. Templates to measure this angulation are available in the marketplace or can simply be fashioned from cardboard in the laboratory.

The setup described in chapter 9 uses the Condyloform II posterior tooth (Candulor), which is based on the lingualized occlusion concept according to Gerber. For this reason, the following steps of the model analysis are based on this principle, omitting both the correction lines as well as angle templates for the stop line.

1. Metric midlines

The metric midlines serve as an orientation line for the subsequent steps of the model analysis (Fig 6-1). **They do not necessarily correspond with the facial midline.** In the maxilla, the incisive papilla and the tuberosities are encircled and quartered with a pencil. With a set square, the distance between the centers of the tuberosities is halved and marked on the palate with a point. This point is connected via a line drawn through the center of the incisive papilla. In the majority of cases, one will observe that this line also runs along the median suture line.

In the mandible, the distance between the centers of the retromolar pads is halved with a set square and marked in the lingual space with a point. The lingual frenulum is used as the anterior reference point and connected with a line.

The lines are extended to the dorsal model margins, and the models are returned to the articulator. When viewed from the dorsal, a large divergence between the metric model midlines can suggest a faulty centric relation record and should be reviewed.

2. Anterior boundaries

In the maxilla, the midpoint of the incisive papilla is now transferred to the lateral model margins; in the mandible, the center of the anterior ridge crest is used. These markings allow for the ideal positioning of the basal aspect of the anterior teeth.

Next, the anterior boundaries are marked. In order to prevent anteroposterior rocking during the incising of food, placement of the incisal edges too far labially must be avoided. In the maxilla, the incisal edges should not be placed more than 7 to 9 mm anterior to the center of the incisive papilla. In the mandible, the lowest point of the labiovestibular fornix forms the boundary. The boundaries are marked with a line on the lateral model borders.

3. Base static lines

The so-called "base static lines" indicate the ideal position for the maxillary supporting cusps and the mandibular central fossae. In the early stages of edentulism, these lines run fairly congruent between both jaws.

As the anterior reference points, the positions of the first premolars are established. The attachment of the buccal frenula as well as the second pair of the palatal rugae are used as references. If neither of these structures is identifiable, the selected anterior card of teeth may be used. The estimated positions of the first premolars are marked with a dot, and the highest contour of the posterior ridges are traced with a pencil held parallel to the tabletop. A

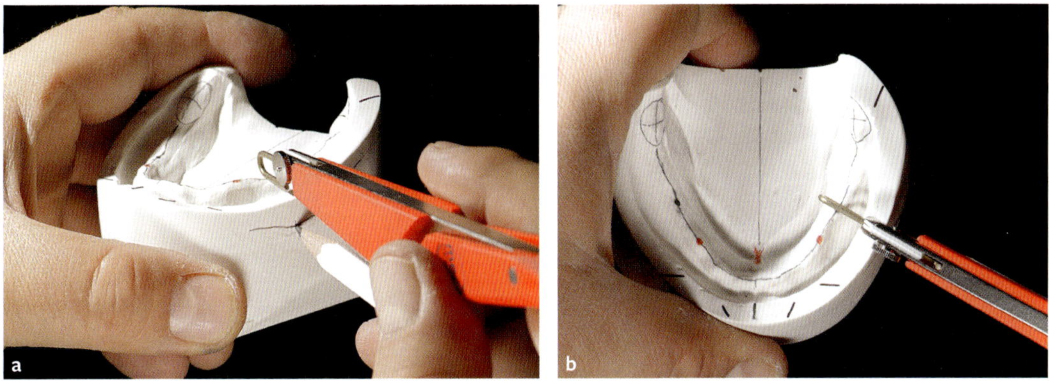

FIG 6-2 (*a*) A profile compass is used to transfer the contours of the residual ridges onto the model base. (*b*) The profile compass must be held parallel to the tabletop and at a strict right angle to the base static line.

straight line reconciling this often slightly curved ridge contour is transferred to the anterior and posterior model margins with a ruler or set square and forms the base static line.

4. Ridge profile

To identify the lowest and highest points of the residual ridges, the sagittal stable zone, and the stop line, a profile compass is used to draw the ridge contours onto the lateral model bases. It is important to hold the guide rod parallel to the occlusal plane and at a right angle to the base static lines (Fig 6-2).

The established lowest point is the ideal position for the largest chewing units, typically the first molars. The same procedure is repeated in the maxilla to determine the highest point.

Both models are then returned into the articulator, and the ridge contours are evaluated. Ideally, the highest and lowest areas are congruent in both arches and the areas about 3 to 4 mm anterior and posterior to the highest and lowest points are parallel to each other and the occlusal plane, or nearly so. If not, a compromise must be found.

The so-determined stable zone forms the masticatory center. A horizontal line is drawn with a pencil, and the lowest point is then marked on the crest of the ridge.

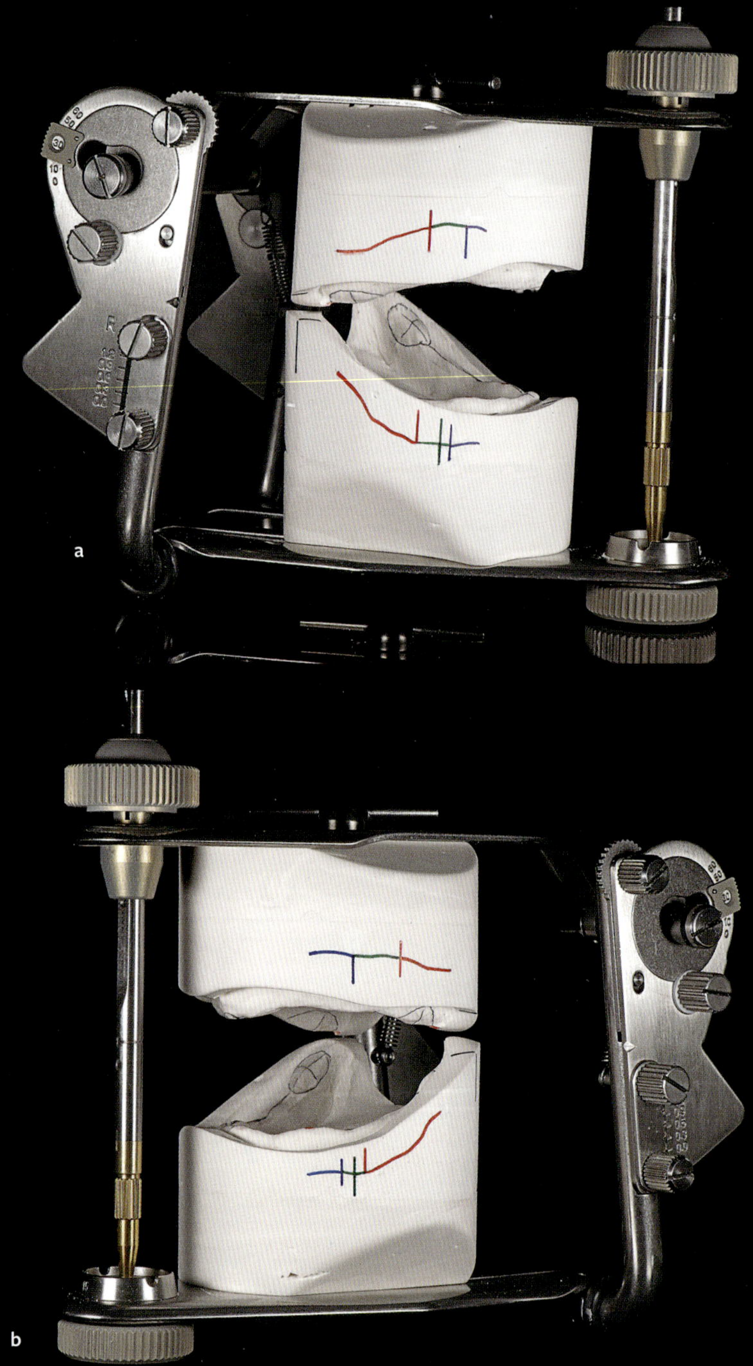

FIG 6-3 (*a and b*) The areas marked in *green* establish the sagittal stable zone. This area contains the lowest point of the residual ridges and, ideally, runs parallel between both arches. The *red line* indicates the stop line. No occlusal contacts must occur distal to this boundary. Note the small stable zone available in this case.

5. Stop line

To avoid the "proglissement," or forward gliding, of the mandibular denture in particular, no masticatory forces must be exerted onto inclined planes such as the ascending ramus of the mandible. The stop line determines the unstable areas. Lerch suggested a maximum incline of 22.5 degrees, while Gerber established a stop line avoiding any incline altogether. Both approaches have merit, depending on the case; however, the author typically uses the stop line as established by Gerber. The area distal to the stop line is considered the unstable zone and is typically marked in red (Fig 6-3).

Conclusion

The goal of the model analysis is to create a visual plan for the setup of artificial teeth. The lowest point in the mandible and the highest point in the maxilla are the ideal positions for the largest masticatory unit, typically the first molars. In many cases, a crossbite setup can be avoided when opting for a lingualized occlusal concept. However, if the base static lines are offset by more than 80 degrees viewed from dorsal, the posterior teeth must be set in crossbite.

7

ESTHETICS

Dentofacial Harmony

In the previous chapters, the basic steps to achieve an ideal fit, positional stability, and masticatory function were described. However, achieving an ideal esthetic outcome is of equal importance. Dentures and other forms of full-mouth rehabilitation restore much more than the ability to masticate food. The importance of restoring the natural appearance of not just the teeth but the entire face cannot be overstated.

In today's society, lighter shades of teeth with more youthful shapes dominate the patient's desired self-image. This is certainly understandable, and ultimately the patient has the final say when it comes to esthetics. However, this does not absolve the treatment team from serving as a guide and advisor. Hardly any patient will express their desire for an artificial and grotesque-looking prosthesis. Tact and empathy in this context are as important as technical, clinical, and artistic skills.

With the composition of the esthetic zone, the appearance and expression of the patient can be either restored or disfigured. The human being as a whole is comprised of the body, the extremities, and the head, which together form a certain harmony. The teeth as part of this harmony are no exception. To achieve truly esthetic outcomes, the individuality of the patient must not be suppressed but emphasized (Figs 7-1 and 7-2).

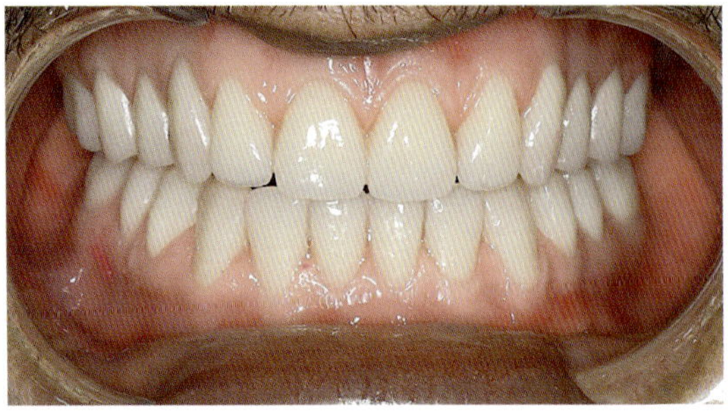

FIG 7-1 An individual arrangement of the anterior teeth helps to create an inconspicuous prosthesis.

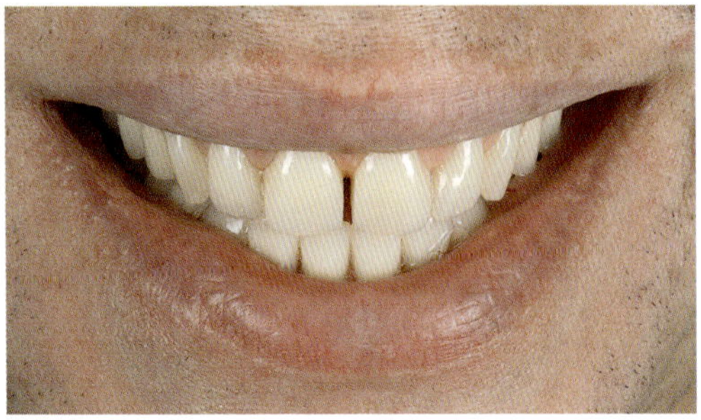

FIG 7-2 To achieve truly esthetic outcomes, the individuality of the patient must not be suppressed but emphasized.

In today's reality, the laboratory technician usually does not get to meet the patient. Laboratory prescription forms may contain the name and perhaps the gender of the patient. With this blatant lack of information, an individually designed restoration can hardly be expected. As such, technicians usually become accustomed to a median-value style of setting teeth.

It must be underscored here again that opinions about what is considered esthetic greatly differ. However, the ultimate esthetic goal of any prosthetic restoration must be to blend in with the patient's appearance. To achieve this, one must consider the age, gender, personality, and physiognomy of the patient. Clinicians are therefore strongly encouraged to provide photography and the results of the esthetic consultation to the technician.

Tooth Shade

Artificial teeth are available in many different shades and nuances today. In natural teeth, the yellowish dentin shimmers through layers of bluish enamel of varying thickness. The incisal edges are generally more translucent and, due to the dark background of the oral cavity, appear grayish blue. Similarly, artificial teeth come in different layers to mimic this interplay of translucency and colors.

The time in which porcelain denture teeth represented the most realistic replacement option for natural teeth is long gone. Multilayered acrylic and composite teeth with their strikingly life-like, vivid appearances are now the norm.

The shade of natural teeth changes throughout the years. The juvenile tooth appears brighter, and the incisal edges are more transparent. With age, the natural teeth begin to darken, partially due to the abrasion of enamel. This naturally occurring change should be considered when selecting the shade for any restoration. Certainly most patients will expect an improvement in shade, but a bleach shade with high incisal translucency and youthful mamelons on an elderly patient will surely be perceived as artificial by their social environment.

The selected shade must match the general appearance of the patient. Here one must consider the color of the skin and hair as well as the white of the eyes. Too stark of a contrast will distract and impart artificiality.

Shape Selection

Many authors have reflected on the correlation between physiognomy and tooth shape in an effort to create a reliable guide for the selection of tooth shapes. Kretschmer's teachings on body types (athletic, leptosome, pyknic), and Williams's theses on the three different shape categories of the face (square, triangular, ovoid) are still used to an extent. In the 1950s, Frush and Fisher developed and propagated the "dentogenetic concept," which considered both facial and intraoral features as well as age, gender, and temperament. While there is no exact way to correlate these physical features reliably with the shape of the teeth, they at least create a starting point.

The creation of a preextraction record via intraoral scan or impression should be considered a standard measure and serve as a reference for any future restoration (Fig 7-3). While it is common that denture teeth are used as they are manufactured, true individuality will be achieved by contouring the prefabricated tooth skillfully to match the given situation.

Gysi observed early on that the dimensions and proportions of the central and lateral incisors correlate with the frontal process of the maxilla and the nasal process. Gerber's research and development of the embryogenetic concept verified these findings. From this it can be asserted that the width of the four maxillary incisors coincides with the width of the piriform aperture. Externally, the width of the anterior six teeth then correlates with the width of the nose from ala to ala (Fig 7-4).

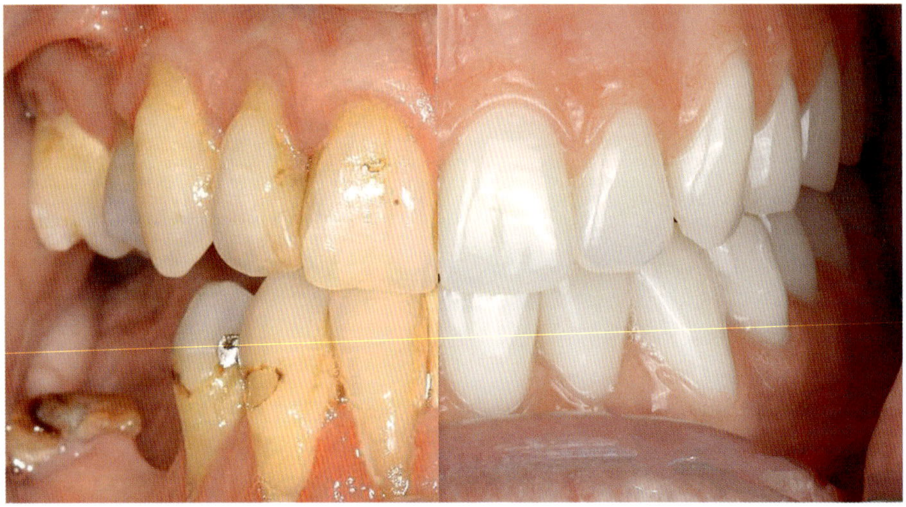

FIG 7-3 The creation of a preextraction record should be considered a standard measure and serve as a reference for any future restoration.

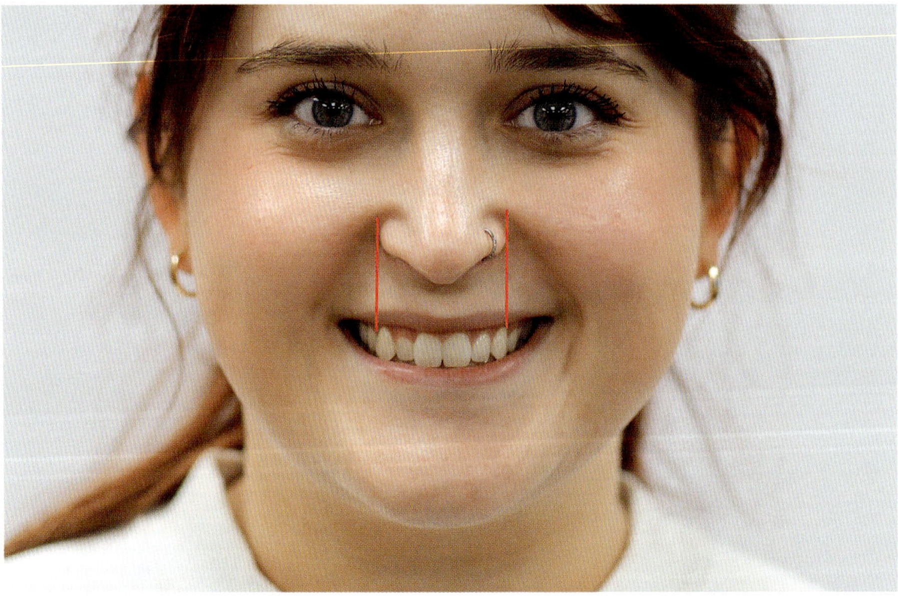

FIG 7-4 The width of the anterior teeth correlates to the width of the nose from ala to ala.

For the selection and placement of the anterior teeth, Gerber discovered basic facts with his teaching of embryogenetics and dentofacial harmony. His considerations and findings assumed that all harmonious structures in

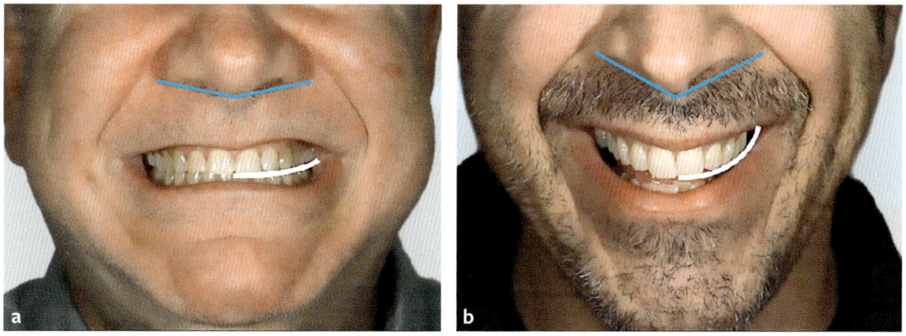

FIG 7-5 (*a*) Relatively flat nasal base and lower lip course. A correspondingly flat anterior arch creates dento-facial harmony. (*b*) With a more sweeping nasal base and lower lip course, the incisal edge line must also run analogously.

animate and inanimate nature are subject to either the laws of crystallization or the laws of cell division, cell differentiation, and segmentation. These laws in conjunction with the embryology of the human face make it possible to determine the proportional ratio of the central and lateral incisors as well as their length ratios. The development and position of the alveolar processes determines the position of the central and lateral incisors and canines.

The frontal and nasal processes, the right and left maxillary processes, and the right and left mandibular processes are involved in the development of the human face. In postnatal development, the embryonic frontal and nasal processes and the associated so-called "intermediate jaw" result in the four maxillary incisors of the primary and permanent dentition. From this it can be concluded that the total width of the four maxillary incisors must be identical to the width of the intermaxilla.

The curve of the anterior arch in relation to the base of the nose is also evident from the embryogenetic analogy according to Gerber. The harmony of a natural anterior arch shows a parallelism with the nasal baseline and the upper edge of the slightly opened lower lip. With a relatively flat nasal base and lower lip course, a flat anterior arch will also fit harmoniously and naturally into the overall picture (see Fig 7-9b). With a more sweeping nasal base and lower lip course, the incisal edge line must also run analogously (Fig 7-5). In narrow, elongated faces, there is often a relatively pointed arch of the base of the nose, which usually corresponds to an equally narrow mouth with a pointed arch of the lower lip.

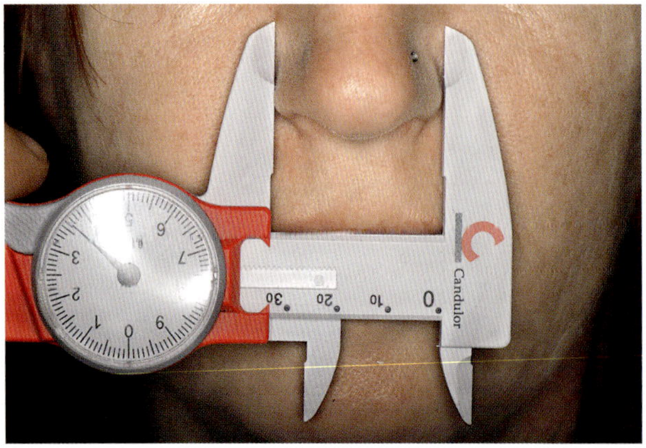

FIG 7-6 As an alternative to the Alameter, a sliding caliper may be used to measure the inter-ala distance.

TRIANGULAR

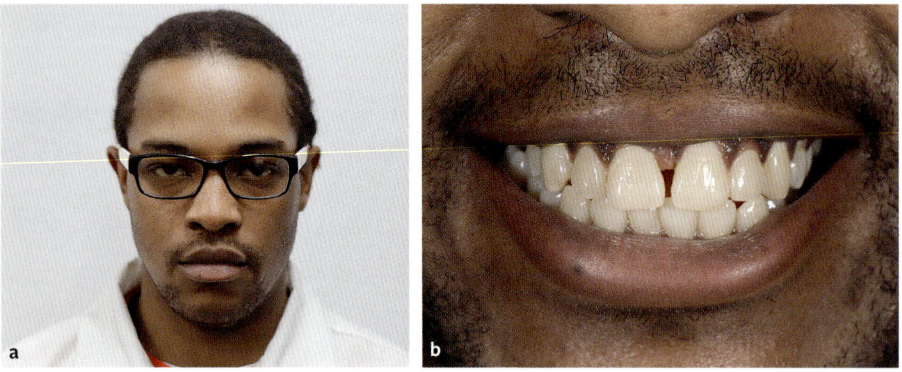

FIG 7-7 (*a*) Triangular face shape. (*b*) Corresponding triangular tooth shape.

Based on these observations, Frush and Lee developed the Alameter. This simple tool is used to measure the distance between the alae and allows for a preselection of maxillary anterior tooth sets. Many tooth manufacturers today provide an Alameter in combination with their respective mould charts. Alternatively, a sliding caliper may be used (Fig 7-6). With a Living Mould Guide (Ivoclar), a final selection of the individual tooth mould can be completed. This final selection should fall within the competence of the clinician or an experienced laboratory technician with access to either the patient or a series of photographs.

Figures 7-7 to 7-10 show various face shapes and their analogous tooth shapes for reference.

OVOID

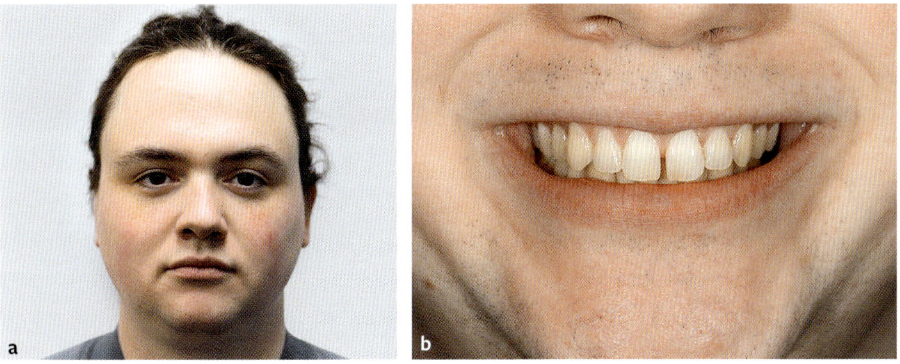

FIG 7-8 (*a*) Ovoid face shape. (*b*) Corresponding ovoid tooth shape.

RECTANGULAR

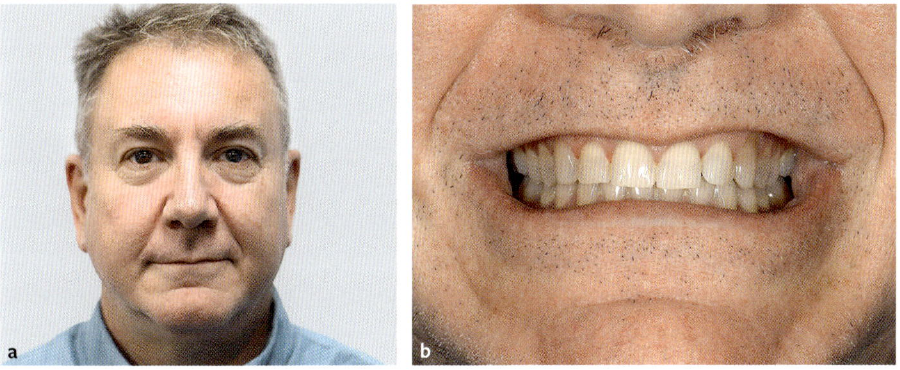

FIG 7-9 (*a*) Rectangular face shape. (*b*) Corresponding rectangular tooth shape.

TAPERING

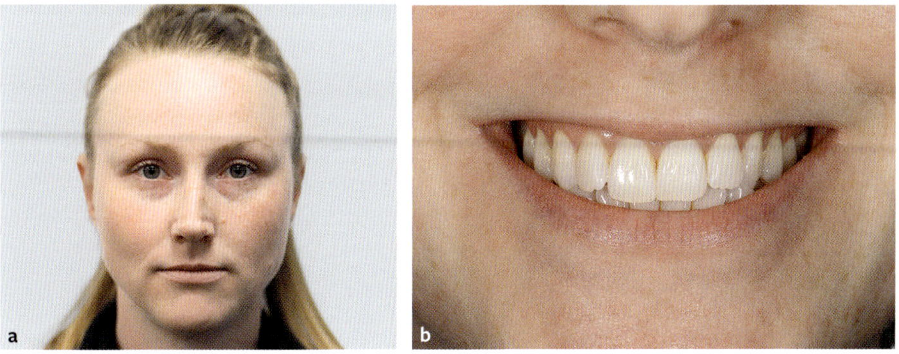

FIG 7-10 (*a*) Slightly tapering face shape. (*b*) Corresponding slightly tapering tooth shape.

Facial Analysis

The adjusted wax rims serve the dental laboratory technician as an esthetic template in terms of incisal edge position, facial midline, lip support, and tooth length. While the general shape of the face can give references for the selection of anterior tooth shape, as shown in Figs 7-7 to 7-10, further valuable information can be found in the analysis of angulations and asymmetries of the patient's face. To create dentofacial harmony, the long axes of the incisors should describe a continuation of these asymmetries, while the frontal long axes of the canines should follow the angulation of the sides of the face (Fig 7-11).

The implementation of these findings requires a great deal of artistic intuition and tact. The patient may have different esthetic goals for their restoration, and the clinician and the technician must be empathetic when balancing these wishes and the presenting data.

FIG 7-11 The central and lateral incisors follow the curvature of the nose, philtrum, and chin with their long axes. The angulation of the cheeks gives a reference for the long axes of the canines.

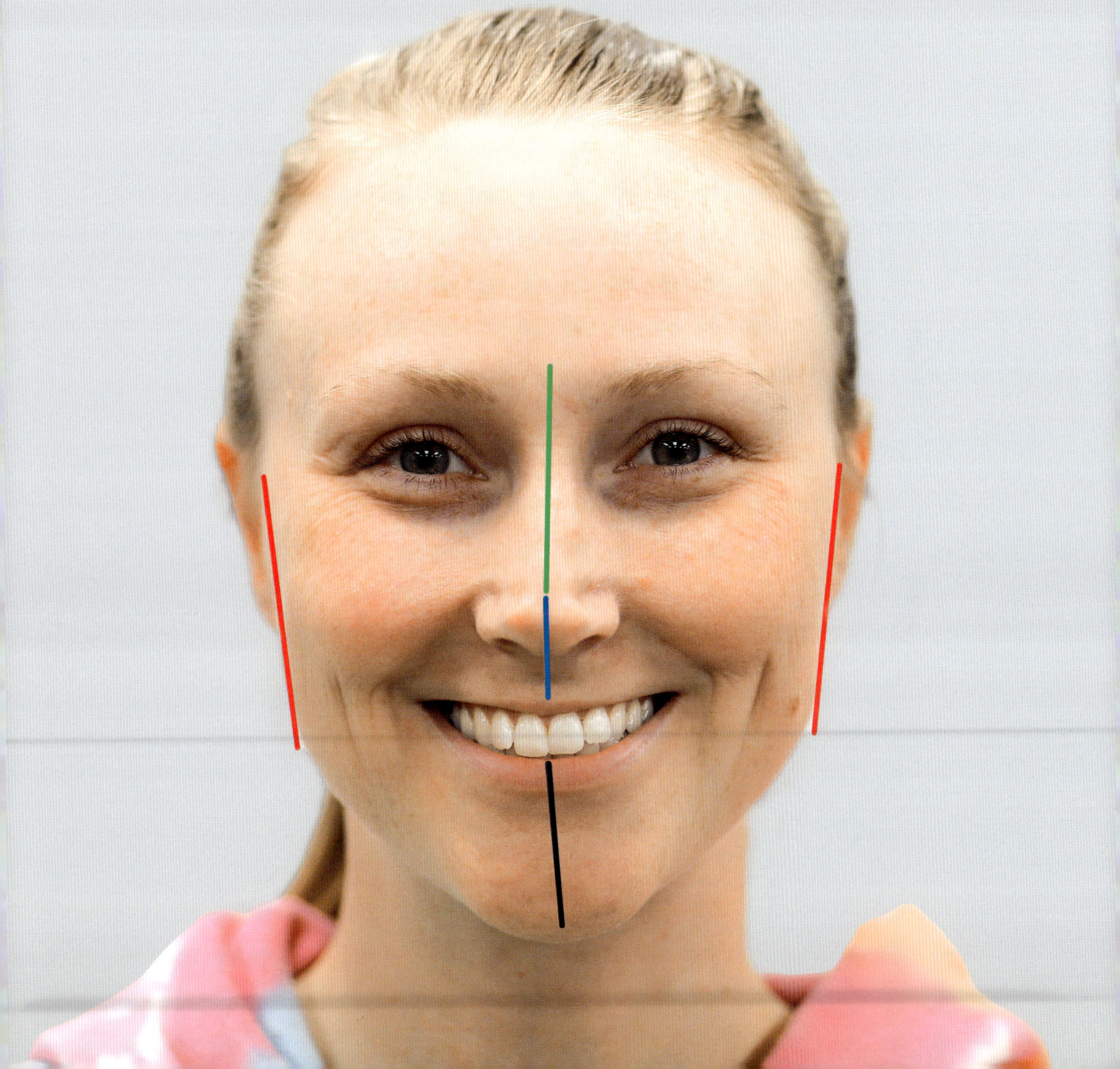

8

ANTERIOR TOOTH SETUP

Composition of the Maxillary Anterior Teeth

The model analysis (see chapter 6) and the patient-specific data recorded by the clinician (see chapter 4), along with good photography, provide the laboratory technician with all the necessary information for an individualized composition of the anterior teeth (Fig 8-1). A facial analysis is used to reveal asymmetries of the face, which should extend into the anterior composition to achieve dentofacial harmony (see chapter 7).

Depending on the method used to mount the models, a flat setup table (when working without a facebow) or a putty matrix (when working with a facebow) is used to preserve the incisal length, labial position, and midline of the central incisors (Fig 8-2).

Generally, the technician will start by setting up the maxillary central incisors (Fig 8-3). The incisal edges should point in an imagined arc toward the lowest point of the mandibular labial vestibule (Fig 8-4).

The maxillary lateral incisor is placed next to the central incisors (Fig 8-5). With a rotation mesial or distal along the long axis, the facial display of the tooth can be increased or reduced. Facial asymmetries can be corrected with the lateral incisors (Fig 8-6).

The individual step between the incisal edges of the central and lateral incisors should be determined by mediating the contour of the base of the nose (alae, columella) and the course of the lower lip when smiling.

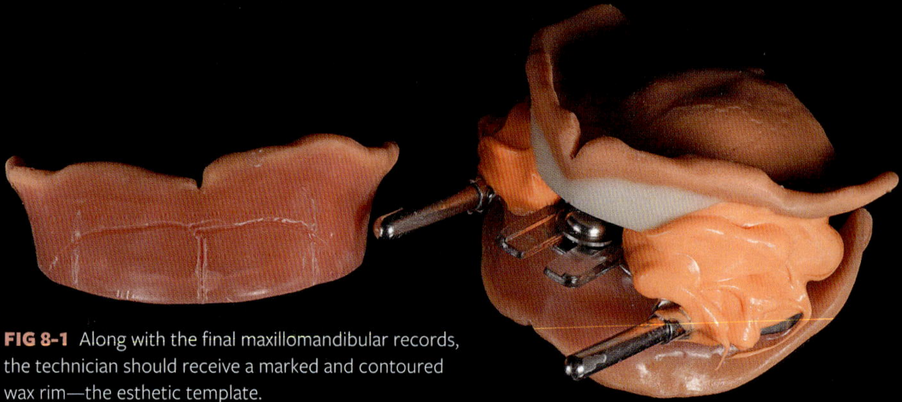

FIG 8-1 Along with the final maxillomandibular records, the technician should receive a marked and contoured wax rim—the esthetic template.

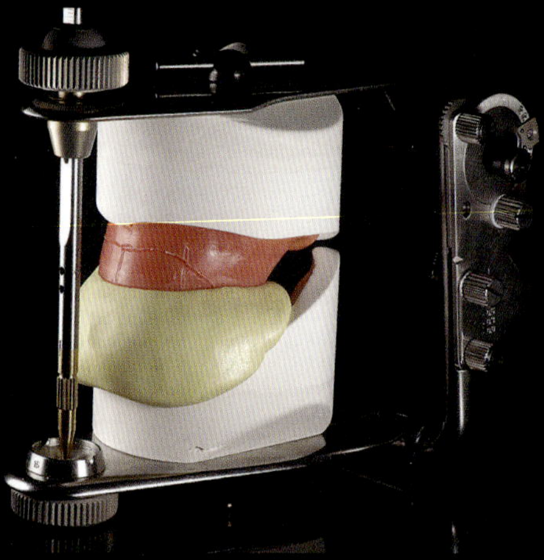

FIG 8-2 A putty matrix preserves the esthetic parameters of the wax rim.

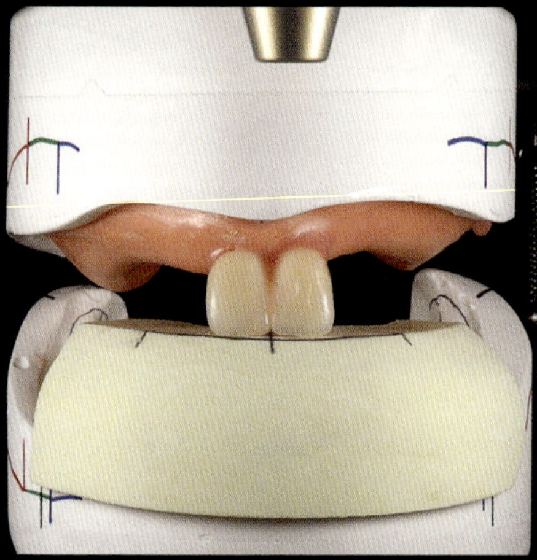

FIG 8-3 The incisal edges of the central incisors are oriented to the matrix.

Next, the maxillary canines are positioned based on the markings of the alae provided by the clinician (Fig 8-7). From an occlusal view, the distal incisal edges of the canines must be oriented toward the base static line (see chapter 6). Viewed from the front, the distofacial facets of the canines should not be visible. The cervical third of the canines stands further buccal than the tip. The buccal tooth axis is perpendicular to the occlusal plane.

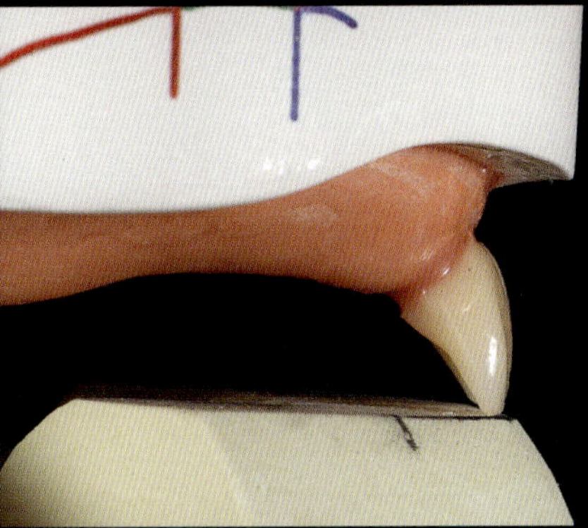

FIG 8-4 The incisal edge of the maxillary central incisor points in an imaginary arc toward the mandibular labial vestibule. In general, the central incisor lies approximately 7 to 9 mm in front of the center of the incisal papilla.

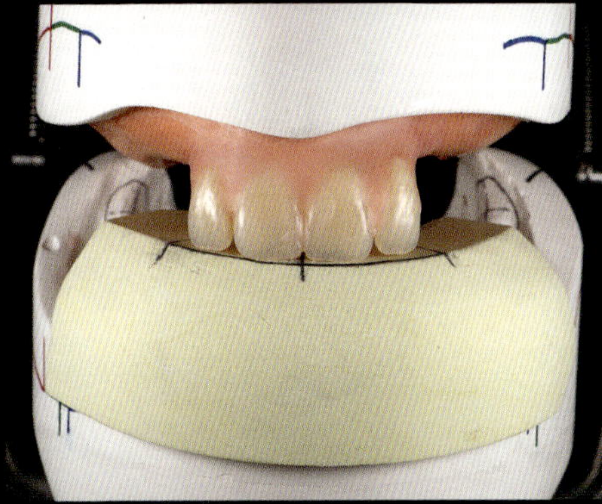

FIG 8-5 The lateral incisors are set between 0.5 and 1.5 mm shorter than the central incisors.

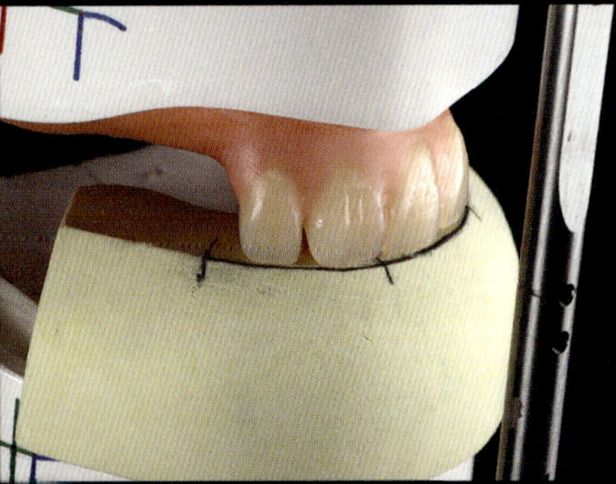

FIG 8-6 Facial asymmetries can be corrected with the lateral incisors.

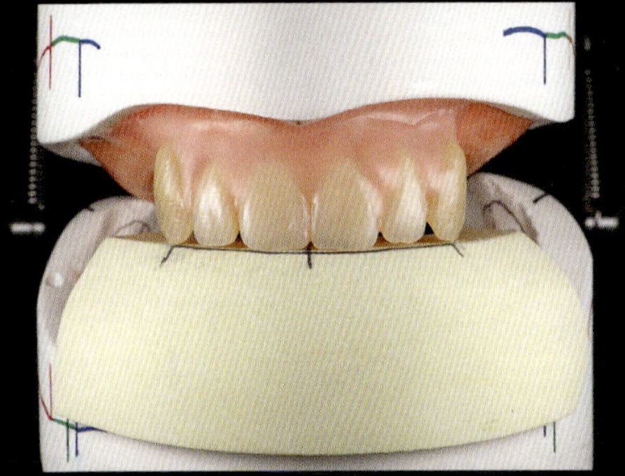

FIG 8-7 The alignment of the canines orients itself to the angulation of the face.

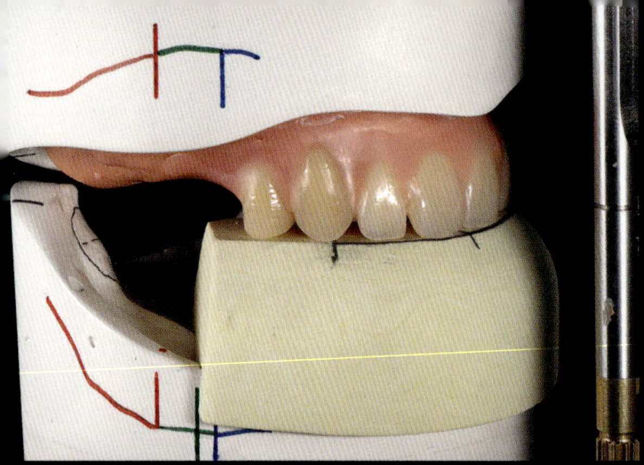

FIG 8-8 Preliminary setup of the maxillary first premolars.

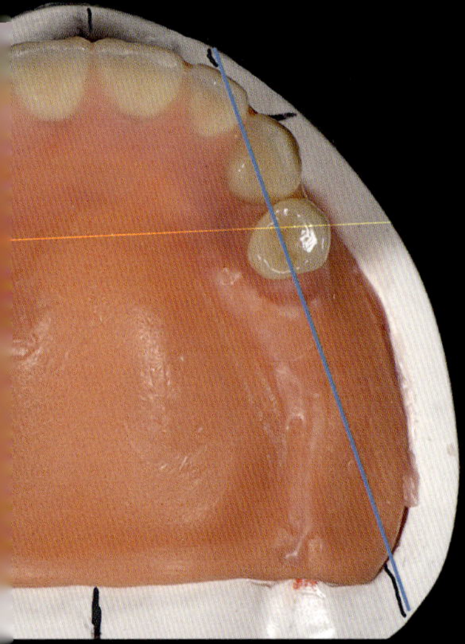

FIG 8-9 The first premolar's central mesial fossa lies above the base static line.

The maxillary anterior setup concludes with a preliminary setup of the maxillary first premolars (Fig 8-8). Their central mesial fossa lies above the base static line (Fig 8-9), with both buccal and palatal cusps at the same level (Fig 8-10). The length is oriented to the canines but should be approximately 1 mm below the occlusal plane.

Note: A flat setup table may only be used as an aid for the arrangement of the maxillary anterior teeth and the first premolars in order to ensure parallelism to the occlusal plane. If the models are mounted with a facebow, the setup table cannot be used!

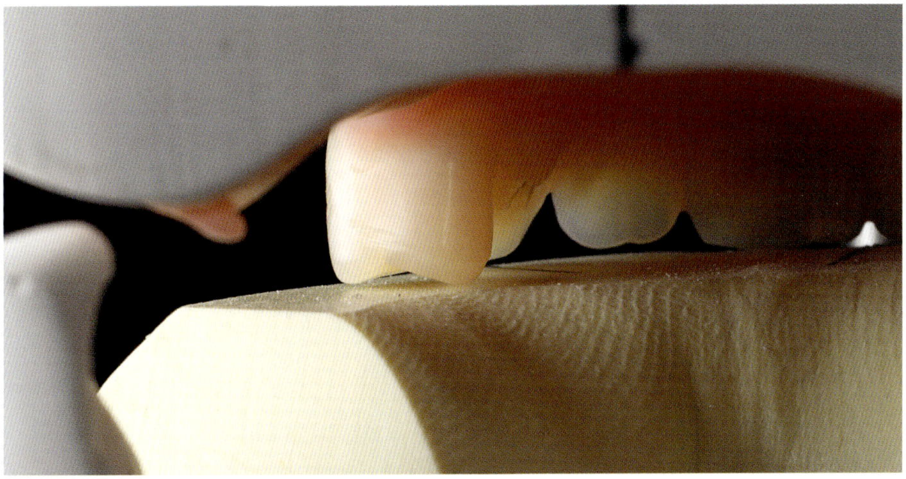

FIG 8-10 The buccal and palatal cusps of the maxillary first premolar are at the same level.

Composition of the Mandibular Anterior Teeth

The arrangement of the mandibular anterior teeth begins with the central incisors. While the often-quoted rule of "1 mm overjet = 1 mm overbite" has validity in Angle Class I cases, the individual overjet and overbite ratio is determined on a case-by-case basis.

While the maxillary anterior teeth are predominantly arranged based on esthetics and phonetics, the mandibular incisors are set with the proximal long axis on the crest of the ridge and a minimal anterior flare. The incisal edges may not protrude further than the lowest point of the labial vestibular fold. Once the mandibular central incisors are set, the condylar elements of the articulator are unlocked, and a protrusive movement of about 3 mm is performed until the incisal edges of the maxillary and mandibular central incisors are atop one another ("crossover"). A slight lifting of the incisal pin from its guide table is desired to allow for later equilibration at the remounting stage.

Note: If an individual sagittal condyle path has been provided, the articulator must be programmed accordingly. Otherwise, the condylar elements are set to a 30-degree average value bilaterally.

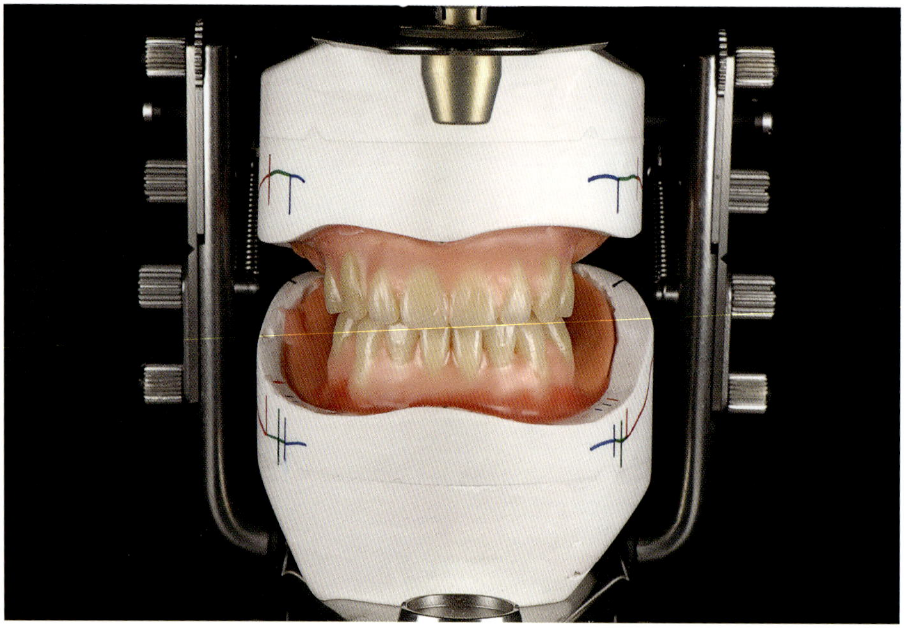

FIG 8-11 Completed anterior composition with the mandibular first premolar added.

This determines and verifies the amount of overjet and overbite for each individual case. After the protrusive check, the condylar elements are locked again.

The mandibular lateral incisors are set analogous to the central incisors but nearly straight in their proximal long axis. While the incisal edges of the mandibular incisors lie with the occlusal plane, the mandibular cuspids are set approximately 1 mm above the plane. Depending on the arrangement of the maxillary cuspids, any canine guidance in laterotrusion will be eliminated during the final equilibration. Similar to the maxillary canines, the cervical third of the mandibular canines stands further buccal. The tooth axis is perpendicular to the occlusal plane.

Figure 8-11 shows a completed anterior tooth setup, including the mandibular first premolars.

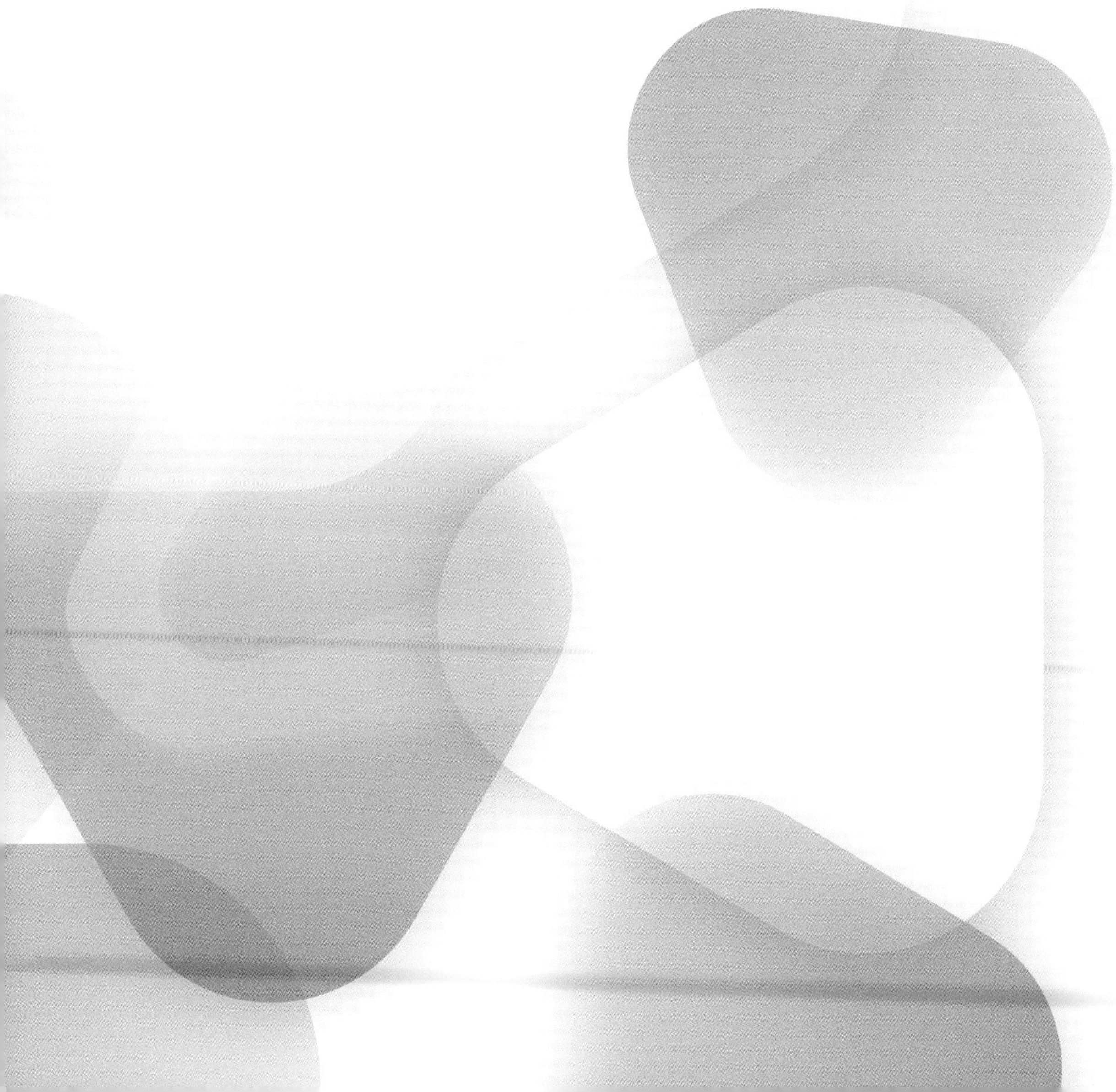

9

POSTERIOR TOOTH SETUP

Occlusal Schemes for Dentures

The goal of positional stability under function and masticatory efficiency presupposes a critical examination of occlusal themes. A simple imitation of natural dentition in terms of position and morphology is insufficient and can lead to dislodgement, discomfort, and damage to the denture-bearing structures—or even to supporting implants.

A fully anatomical posterior tooth with steep and youthful cusps may look beautiful to the morphology afficionado but will hardly be positionally stable in a solely mucosa-supported prosthesis. Any hyperbalances caused by steep cusp slopes and marginal ridges will result in a redirection of force under function, which in turn causes a small dislodgement. In the short term, this effect will lead to discomfort and repeated sore spots, and in the long term it may lead to accelerated atrophy of the residual ridge. Likewise, implant-retained overdentures may suffer from premature wear of the attachment elements. In a worst-case scenario, repeated horizontal thrusting forces may loosen the implants themselves.

Balanced Occlusion

The term *balanced occlusion* can generally be divided into two concepts: *(1)* fully balanced and *(2)* bilaterally balanced.

The aim of a fully balanced occlusion is to support the prostheses during dynamic occlusion in the posterior regions AND in the anterior tooth regions. This concept was developed at a time of non–suction-effective vulcanized rubber dentures and enabled the patient to press both dentures evenly against the supporting tissues to achieve stability. This total prosthesis occlusion concept is associated with the articular theory according to Gysi.

In contrast, the bilaterally balanced occlusion concept serves to exclude contacts in the anterior tooth area during the laterotrusion movement of the mandible. This concept of occlusion avoids the prying effects and shear loads acting on the frontal jaw ridges under anterior tooth contact.

While contemporary occlusal schemes may also include canine guidance or sequential guidance, bilaterally balanced occlusion still represents a sensible approach to reduce or eliminate any tipping or thrusting forces during idle mastication and swallowing. The reader is reminded, however, that **any occlusion is canceled once a food bolus is introduced**, typically unilaterally.

Therefore, a ridge-adequate setup must also be achieved in order to stabilize the dentures during the initial stages of the chewing act, where contacts between the opposing teeth are canceled by the food bolus. This means that all occlusal contacts—centric and dynamic—occur within the stable zone established with the model analysis. This approach also typically places the teeth within the muscular equilibrium.

Remember Gerber's concept of autonomous chewing stability (see chapter 6):

- Each pair of opposing posterior teeth does not destabilize the denture under occlusal load.
- All masticatory forces are directed in their entirety perpendicular to the denture-bearing area.
- No occlusal contacts occur on inclined planes.

Lingualized Occlusion According to Gerber

Given that a large majority of denture cases present with moderately preserved to severely absorbed residual ridges, it makes sense to dispense with the use of fully anatomical teeth. Conversely, monoplane occlusion with no cusps likely will not lead to effective mastication.

In previous chapters, the prerequisites for a symbiotic prosthetic restoration that integrates into the stomatognathic system have been described. To ensure positional stability even under masticatory load, Gerber developed the condylar theory. His approach to lingualized occlusion creates a sound and highly functional prosthesis.

In a 2006 pilot study, Kimoto et al compared the masticatory function, retentiveness, and overall satisfaction of 28 edentulous patients. Half were provided dentures with bilaterally balanced occlusion, and the other half were provided dentures with lingualized occlusion. Despite limitations of this study attributed to the small sample size and lack of randomization, the authors found that edentulous patients fitted with complete dentures with lingualized occlusion experienced and expressed greater satisfaction with their denture retention.

Lingualized occlusion is an often-misunderstood concept. By taking the buccal cusps (A-contacts) out of occlusion, destabilizing contacts buccal to the residual ridge are eliminated. Gerber further designed denture teeth with the mandibular central fossa shifted to the lingual. With the exception of the first premolars, the occlusion is reduced to prominent palatal cusps and simplified fossae in the mandible. An additional equilibration at the remount stage creates freedom in centric occlusion with polyvalent occlusal geometry. This contributes to autonomous chewing stability while also improving cheek support and tongue space.

The Condyloform II Teeth

The consideration of functional, anatomical, and age-related properties as well as the use of high-quality materials are crucial for the success of esthetic and effective dentures. With this in mind, the Condyloform II posterior teeth (Candulor) were developed in close cooperation with the University of Zurich to create a perfect combination of a proven design and new materials.

The second generation of the Condyloform teeth is fabricated from a nanofilled composite material that has proven itself with its excellent wear resistance. The occlusal surfaces are designed according to the mortar-pestle principle (Gerber) and are arranged in a tooth-to-tooth relationship. This principle is based on a morphologic reversal of the temporomandibular joint. The design secures the horizontal jaw relation sufficiently, while reducing the size of the occlusal field, yet allows for increased freedom in centric occlusion, thereby avoiding unnecessary hyperbalances and thrusts.

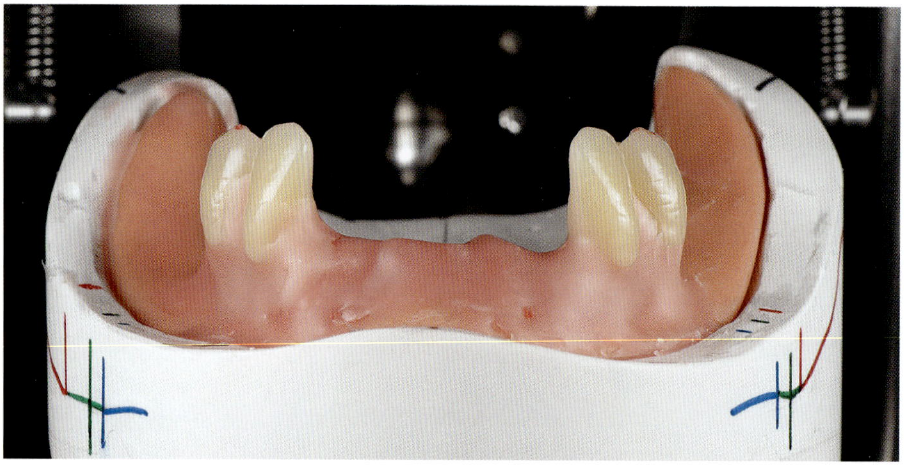

FIG 9-1 The buccal cusps of the mandibular first premolars are set on the occlusal plane, with the lingual cusps approximately 0.5 to 1 mm below the occlusal plane.

In the maxilla, the pestle (microcondyle) is represented by the dominant palatal cusps of the second premolars and the molars. In the mandible, the mortar (microfossa) is formed by a simplified occlusal design with a wide central fossa shifted to the lingual. This microcondyle/microfossa principle creates contact only between a palatal cusp and an antagonist fossa. Contacts between the buccal cusps, with the exception of the first premolars, are eliminated.

The Mandibular Posterior Setup

The first posterior tooth to be set up in the mandible is the first premolar. Its prominent buccal cusp must occlude in the mesial central fossa of the previously set maxillary first premolar. The buccal cusp tip should correspond with the occlusal plane, while the lingual cusp may be 0.5 to 1 mm below the occlusal plane (Fig 9-1). The centric contact is checked and marked with red occlusion ribbon (Fig 9-2). Once the tooth is set, a laser pointer is used

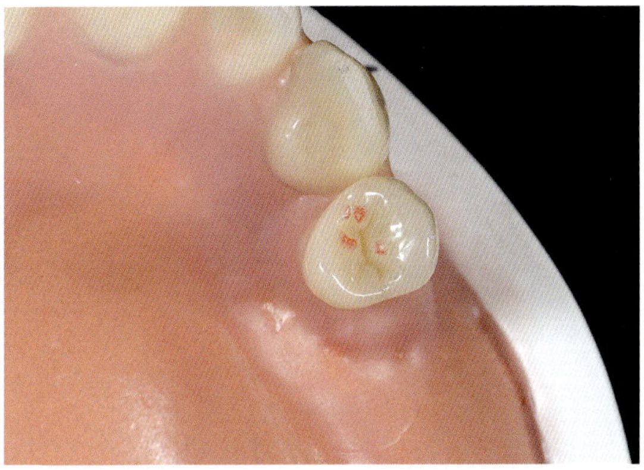

FIG 9-2 The prominent buccal cusp of the mandibular first premolar occludes into the mesial central fossa of the maxillary first premolar in a tripodized pattern.

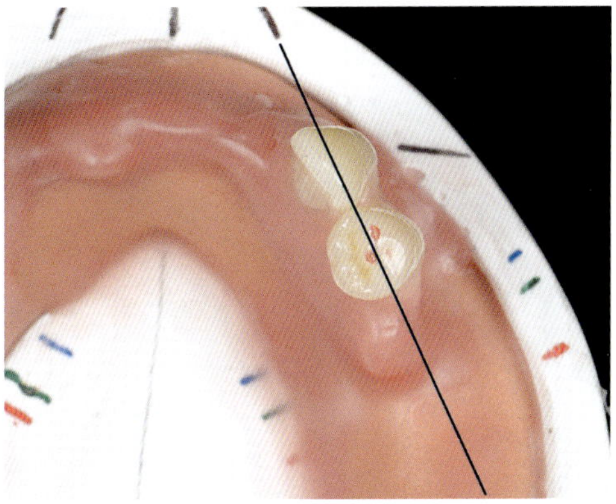

FIG 9-3 The centric contacts lie above the base static line.

to check the relation of the centric contact to the residual ridge. It should be positioned right above the base static line (Fig 9-3).

At this point it may be necessary to make corrections to the preliminary setup of the maxillary first premolar; this is often the result of a narrower mandibular arch. The correction may be done by resetting the maxillary first premolar slightly palatal or, in borderline cases, by moving the mesial fossa palatal via selective grinding.

If the evaluation of the model analysis allows, the mandibular second premolar is then set next to the first premolar. The mandibular second premolar's central fossa is set above the base static line, with both the buccal and lingual cusps level and 0.5 to 1 mm below the occlusal plane.

In the example case shown here, the second premolar is omitted. The mandibular first molar, as the largest chewing unit, is set at the lowest point of the residual ridge, with its central fossa on the base static line as determined by the model analysis (Fig 9-4). Both the buccal and lingual cusps lie on the occlusal plane. Again, the position is checked with a laser pointer.

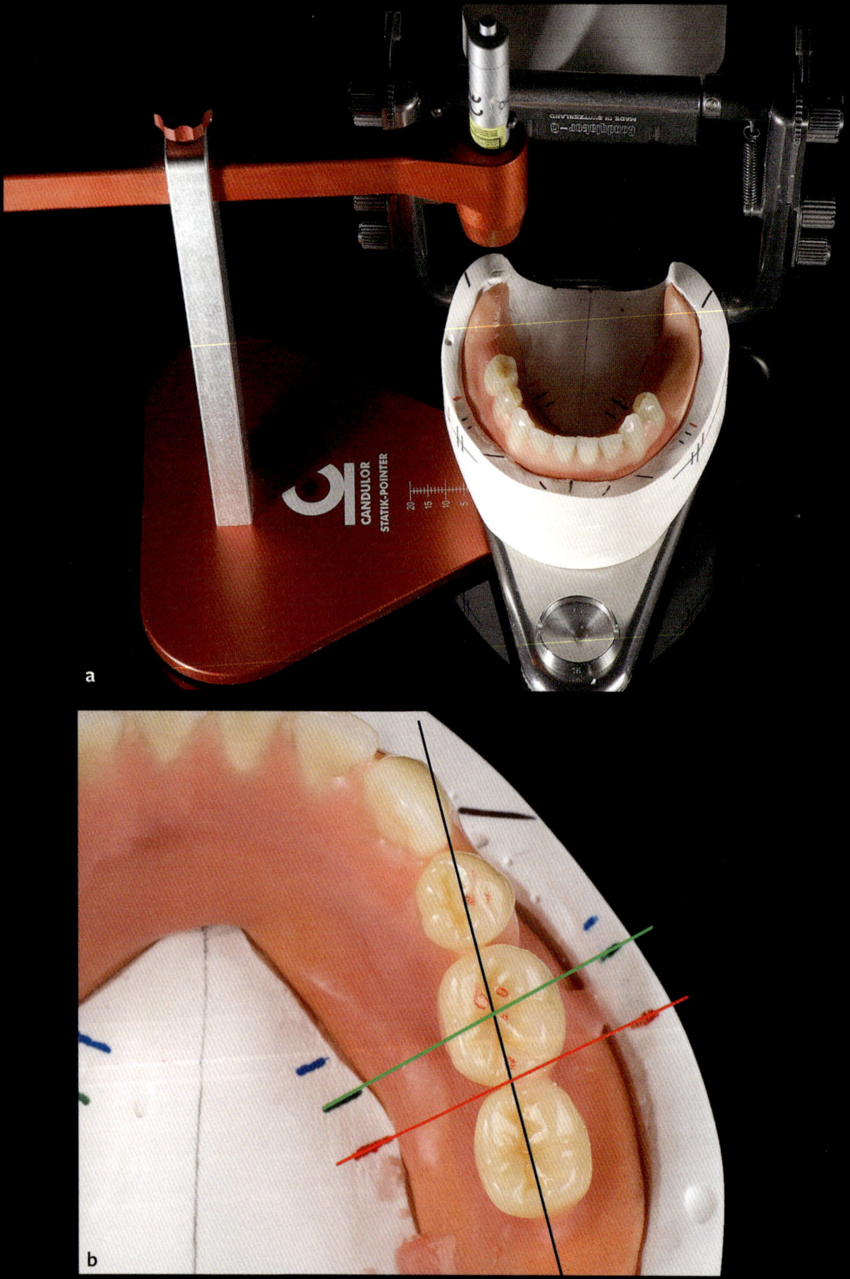

FIG 9-4 (*a and b*) The mandibular first molar, as the largest chewing unit, is set at the lowest point of the residual ridge (*green*), with its central fossa on the base static line (*black*). Note how the anatomical conditions create a shortened row of teeth. The second premolar is omitted, and the second molar lies distal to the stop line and may not be occlusally loaded.

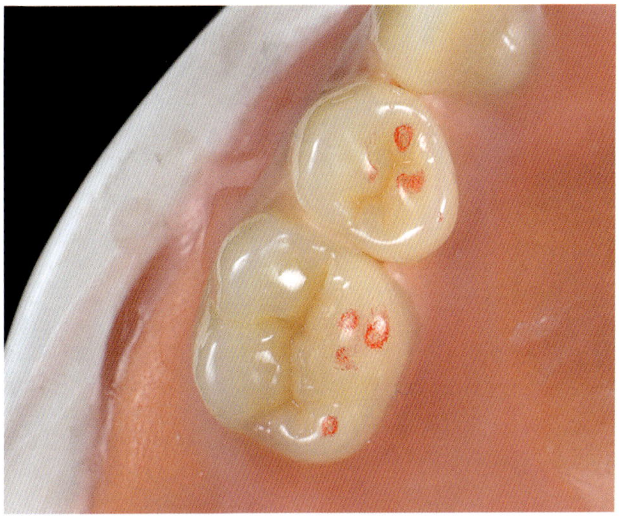

FIG 9-5 The tripod pattern on the mesiopalatal cusp of the maxillary first molar is visible along with a single contact of the distopalatal cusp with the distal marginal ridge of the mandibular first molar.

Finally, the mandibular second molar is set. As the terminal tooth, its mesiobuccal and mesiolingual cusps lie at the occlusal plane, while the distobuccal and distolingual cusps are positioned slightly above the occlusal plane. This creates the sagittal compensation curve that will later allow for the creation of balancing contacts in protrusion.

A pronounced curve in the sense of a sphere of Monson is not required with the Condyloform II posterior teeth.

> **Note: If the model analysis indicates a shortened row of teeth and the mandibular first molar is the terminal tooth, it must be set analogous to the mandibular second molar as described above.**

The Maxillary Posterior Setup

Because the maxillary first premolar is already in its final position, the first tooth to be set is the maxillary first molar. Its prominent mesiopalatal cusp occludes with the central fossa of the mandibular first molar in a tripod pattern (Fig 9-5).

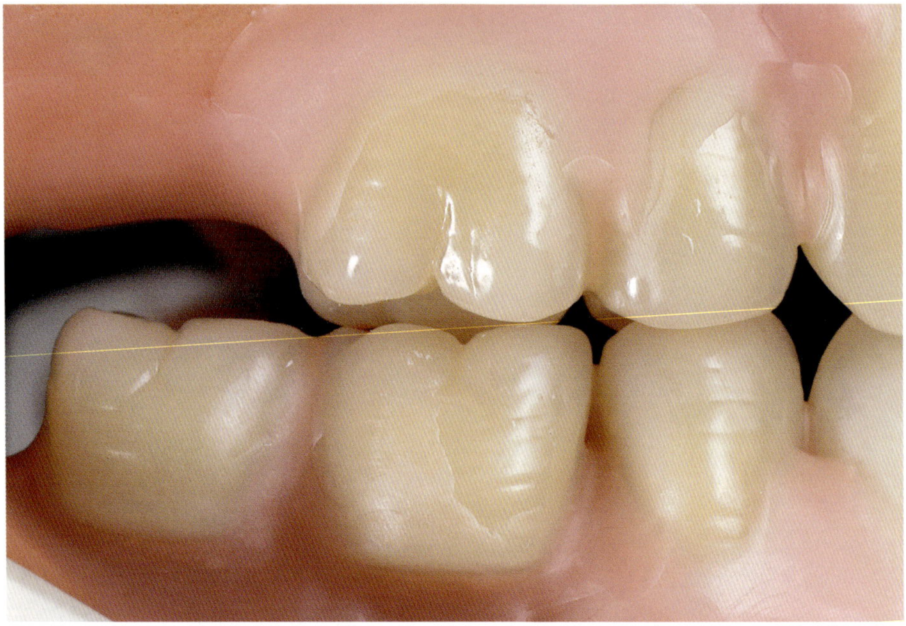

FIG 9-6 With the exception of the first premolar, note the absence of buccal contacts.

The smaller distopalatal cusp occludes with the distal marginal ridge of the mandibular first molar. Note that **the buccal cusps do not occlude** (Fig 9-6).

Next, the maxillary second premolar is set with its palatal cusp occluding with the central fossa of the mandibular second premolar. Again, a tripodized contact pattern is to be achieved. The buccal cusps do not occlude.

If the mandibular second molar has been set, the maxillary second molar is set with its mesiopalatal cusp occluding with the central fossa of the mandibular second molar. Figure 9-7 shows the finalized setup.

It is advisable to not heat the setup wax excessively; the hotter the wax, the stronger the contraction as it cools. Alternating between the quadrants can save time during the setup. Once the setup is completed and the wax has been allowed to cool, all centric contacts must be checked once more with red occlusion ribbon, and their position must be verified against the base static lines established during the model analysis.

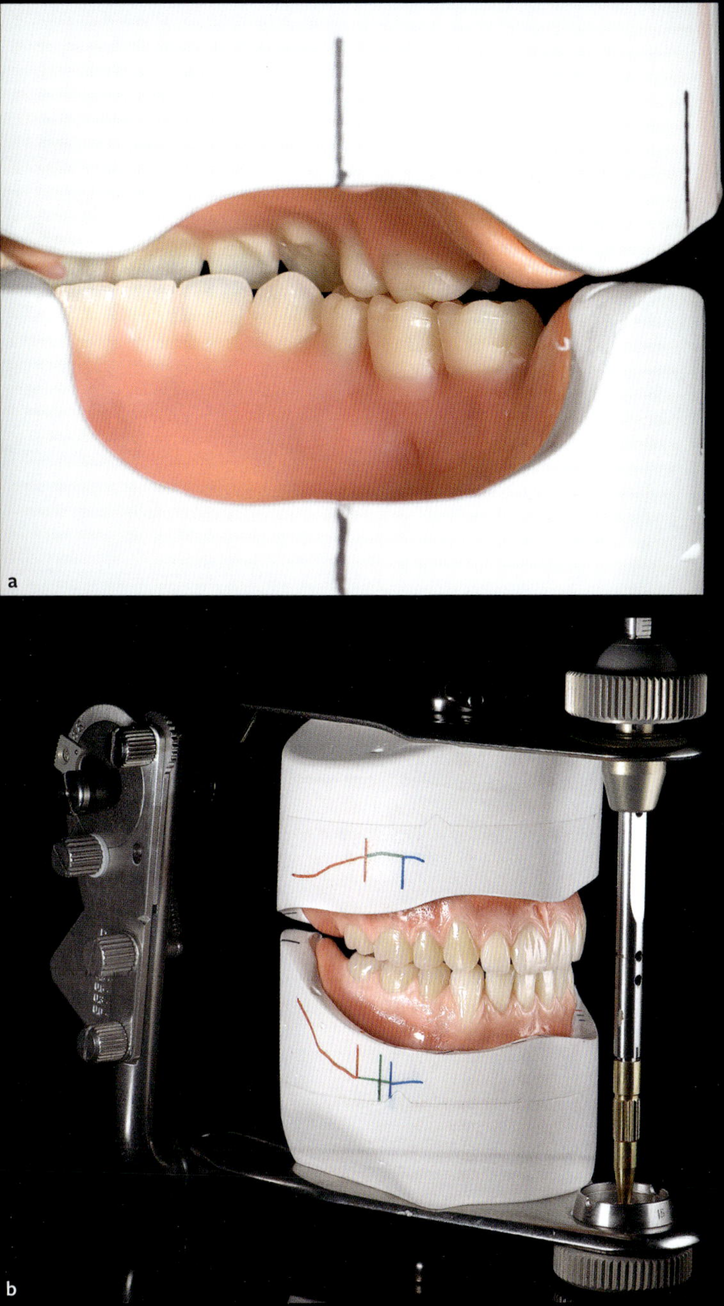

FIG 9-7 (*a*) Lingual view of the posterior tooth setup. (*b*) Finalized setup. Because the second molars are distal to the stop line, the maxillary second molar is set 2 mm out of occlusion and serves only as cheek support.

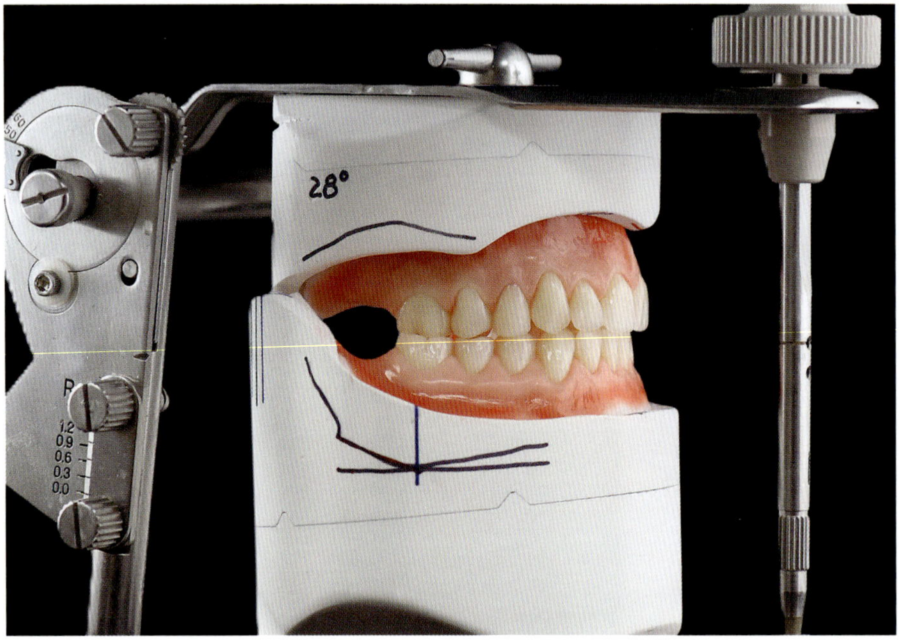

FIG 9-8 This setup uses the second premolar as the transition tooth into a crossbite. In this case, the mandibular second premolar is adjusted to accommodate the buccal and palatal cusps of the maxillary second premolar in an end-to-end fashion. The first molars are in proper crossbite relation.

Crossbite Setup

If a posterior crossbite setup is unavoidable, it is useful in terms of patient acceptance to begin the transition into the crossbite with the second premolars. The mandibular posterior tooth setup begins as described previously, but the maxillary second premolar is set in a cusp-to-cusp relationship. Both the buccal and lingual cusps of the mandibular second premolar are selectively ground to create two small areas into which the buccal and palatal cusps of the maxillary second premolar may occlude. The first molars are set in a proper crossbite intercuspation, with the maxillary buccal cusps occluding with the mandibular central fossae (Fig 9-8).

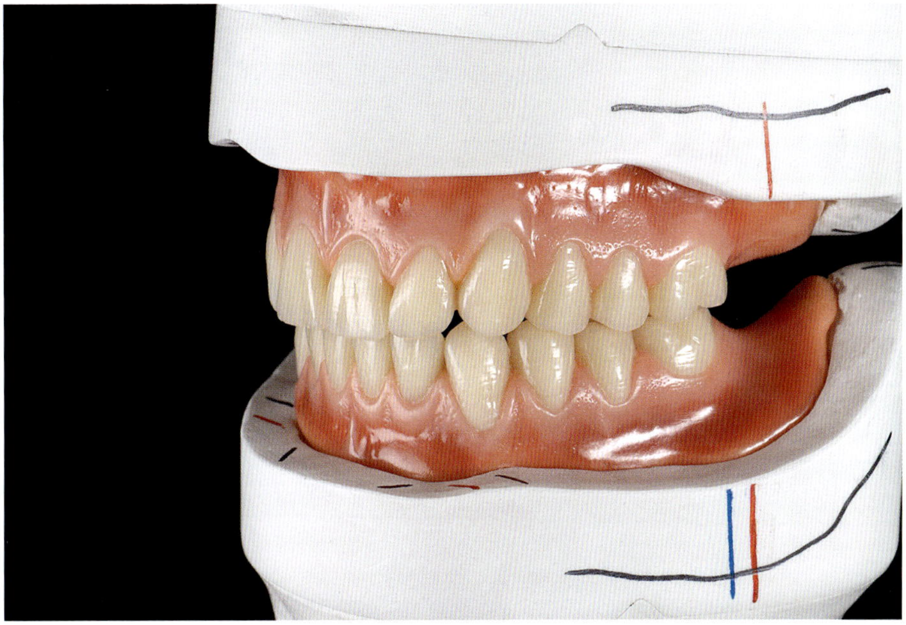

FIG 9-9 Typical arrangement. The second molars are omitted due to the position of the stop line.

Difficult Interalveolar Relationships

Only rarely do we encounter cases with ideal interalveolar relationships, where all posterior teeth can be safely set in their natural, eugnathic positions and order. Many clinicians and laboratory technicians must free themselves from the belief that all 28 teeth delivered on the tooth cards must also be used in the dentures.

Frequently, the posterior setup allows only for a shortened row of teeth. Most often, the second molars are omitted as they likely violate the stop line established with the model analysis (Fig 9-9). Occasionally, it becomes necessary to skip the second premolars instead in order to be able to place the largest chewing unit onto the lowest point of the residual ridge. Conversely, a third pair of premolars may be added at the expense of the second molars in order to place the largest chewing unit appropriately.

Cases with pronounced Angle Class II and Class III malocclusions will require similar adjustments.

10

MODELING OF THE GINGIVA

Artificial Gingiva

The wax denture delivered for try-in should be an accurate representation of the final contours, and even colors, of the final prosthesis. Creating a generic, simplified wax-up of the denture body and only adding final contours later in acrylic deprives both the clinician and the patient of a true assessment during the try-in appointment. This is unfortunately all too common.

There has been much debate among professionals on how detailed artificial gingiva ought to be designed. The arguments against a true-to-life contour and texture range from hygienic concerns to the necessity altogether. However, a healthy, lifelike appearance of the artificial gingiva is part of the overall esthetics of the denture and is well worth the effort.

A hard carving wax, an electric waxing unit, and a double-tipped carving instrument are used in this step (Fig 10-1).

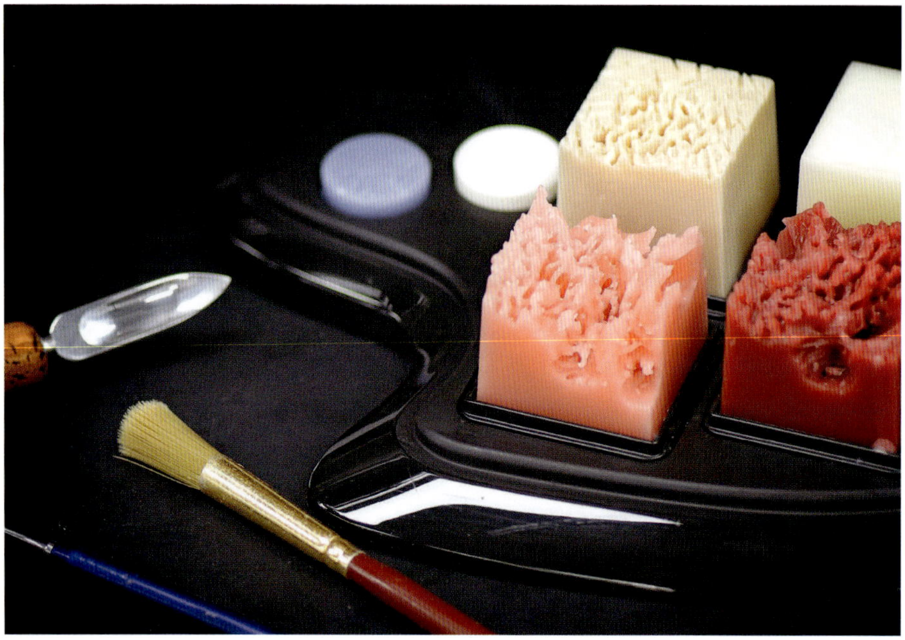

FIG 10-1 A hard carving wax along with an electric waxing unit, a brush, and a sharp, lancet-type carver are all that is required for a realistic wax-up.

Muscular Tactility

Along with esthetic considerations, the functional design of the denture body can have a dramatic impact on the retention of the denture. If implemented correctly, the perioral musculature can form a symbiotic relationship with the denture. While the alveolar mounds are typically of a convex contour, the apical areas are designed more or less concave, up to the drop-shaped contour of the valve margins.

This interplay of convex and concave polished surfaces creates areas to which the perioral muscles can adhere under function (Fig 10-2). This requires the dental technician to have good knowledge of muscular anatomy and function. The main actors to be considered in this context are the orbicularis oris, masseter, buccinator, levator anguli oris, and depressor anguli oris muscles.

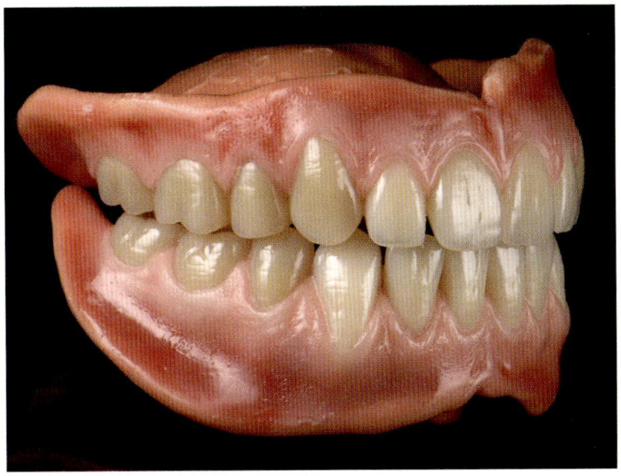

FIG 10-2 An interplay of convex and concave surfaces creates areas to which the perioral muscles can adhere under function.

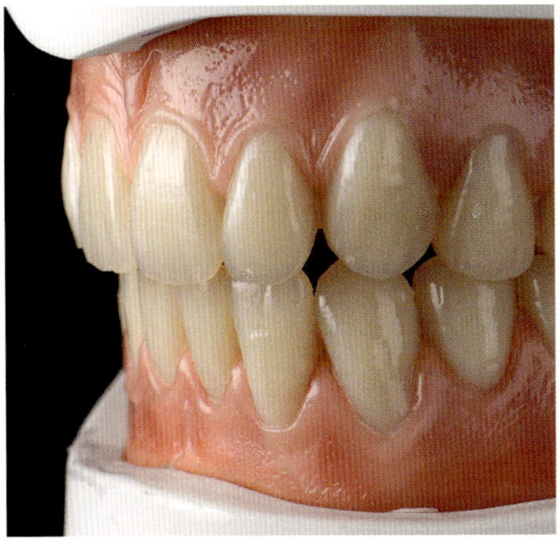

FIG 10-3 The modeling of the lip shield must strike a compromise between hygiene and morphologic realism.

Lip Shield

The (potentially) visible portion of the anterior denture body is called the *lip shield*. It refers to the artificial gingiva typically spanning from first premolar to first premolar. Here the re-creation of natural colors and textures is desired (Fig 10-3). All too often, the artistic inclination of the dental technician can create unhygienic conditions. Avoiding undercuts and deep furrows, which easily collect biomaterials and are difficult to clean, is paramount.

Macroscopically, the lip shield's design follows the morphology of the natural gingiva:

- The free gingiva, which includes the gingival margins and interdental papillae
- The attached gingiva
- The mucogingival junction
- The alveolar mucosa

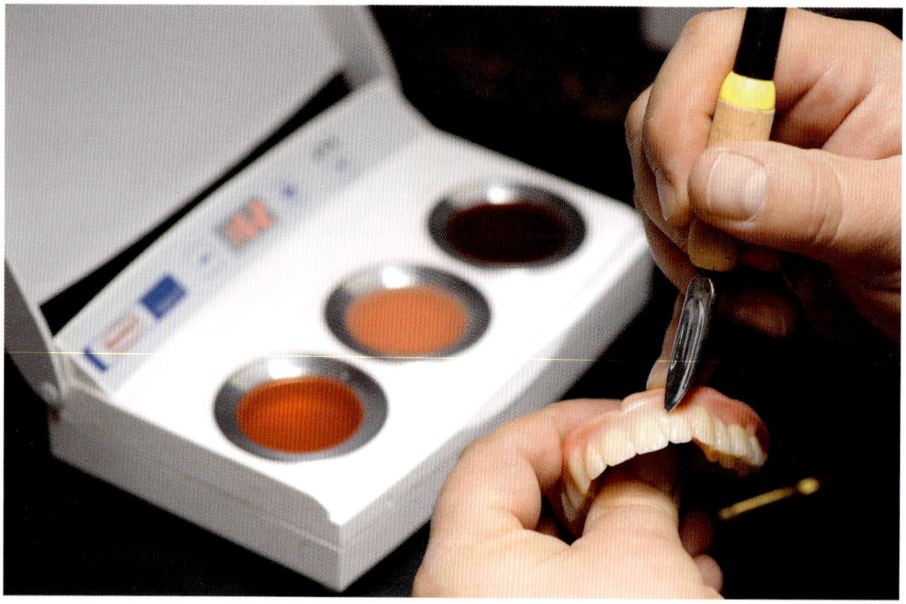

FIG 10-4 Lighter and darker hues of pink can give the illusion of depth.

Modeling in Wax

After completion of the tooth setup, the setup wax must be allowed to fully cool. Any excess setup wax should be removed with a carver or a rotating brush wheel. The valve margins are formed by flowing a medium-hard wax into the vestibular margins of the functional model.

Colored waxes such as GEO Expert Gingiva (Renfert) can be used to great effect. The use of lighter and darker hues of pink can give the illusion of depth without creating unhygienic "niches" (Fig 10-4).

The interdental papillae are best created with a small drop of wax, with the incisal edges facing downward as the wax cools. This way, the cohesion within the wax effortlessly creates a plump, slightly convex contour, which allows food particles to run off instead of becoming trapped in a triangular gap. The gingival margins are carved at an approximate 45-degree angle to the long axis of the tooth using a sharp, lancet-type carver (Fig 10-5).

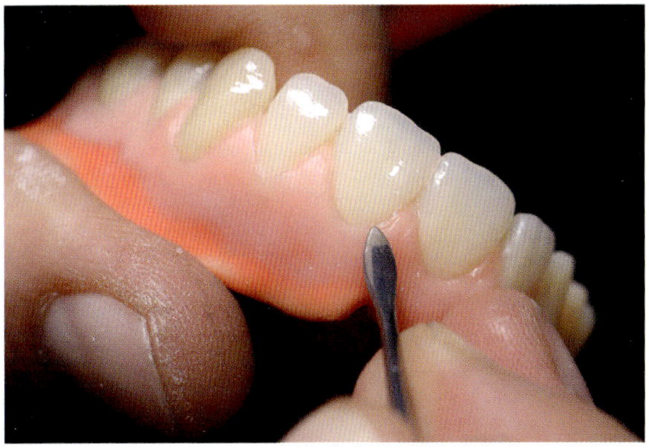

FIG 10-5 The gingival margins are carved at an approximate 45-degree angle to the long axis of the tooth using a sharp, lancet-type carver. Deep furrows are to be avoided.

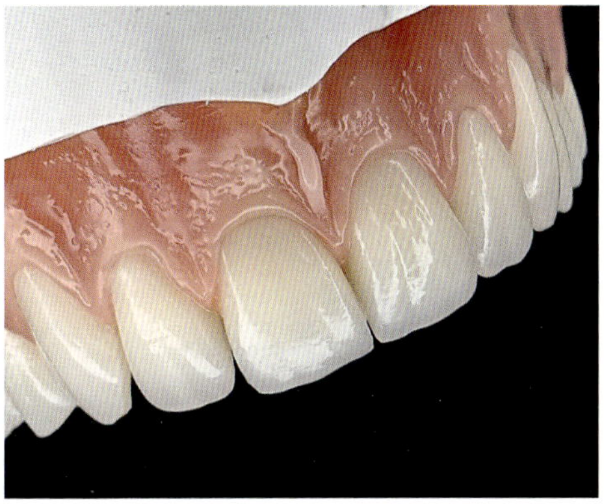

FIG 10-6 The surface textures are softened with an alcohol torch.

Next, the alveolar mounds are created apical to the gingival margins. The mucosa in this area is typically compressed more across the underlying alveoli and appears characteristically "blanched." To recreate this effect, the areas can be accentuated with a light pink or dentin-shaded wax. The areas in between are filled with a richer, reddish wax. The alveolar mucosa usually shows a slight purple hue, which extends toward the valve margins.

The entire wax structure can be covered with a translucent pink wax, depending on the desired intensity of the coloration.

The so-called "stippling effect" occurs only in the area of the attached gingiva. It is a manifestation of the epithelial papillae of the mucosa in this area (lamina propria mucosae). A sponge or soft toothbrush can be used for this purpose. Stippling should always be created in wax; later application in acrylic is nearly impossible to polish and can create hygiene challenges. A gentle smoothing with an alcohol torch is the final step of the wax sculpting (Fig 10-6).

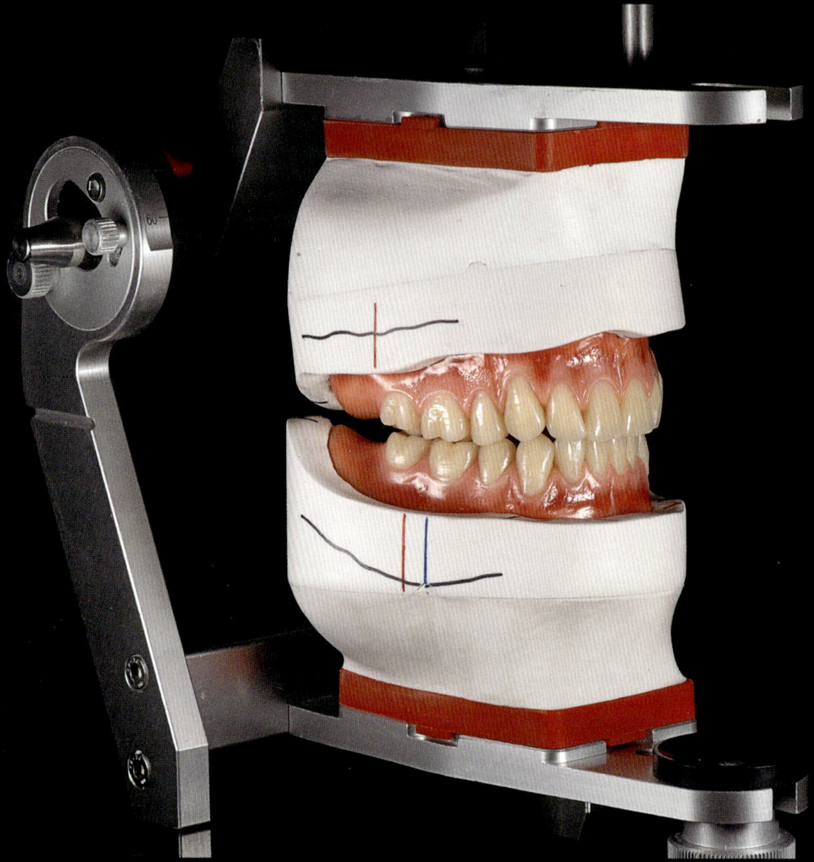

FIG 10-7 After a thorough cleaning, the wax-up is ready for submission to the dentist.

Once the wax-up has been allowed to cool completely, it can be polished further with a cotton ball under cold running water or a few squares of foam plastics mounted in layers onto a screw mandrel (Fig 10-7).

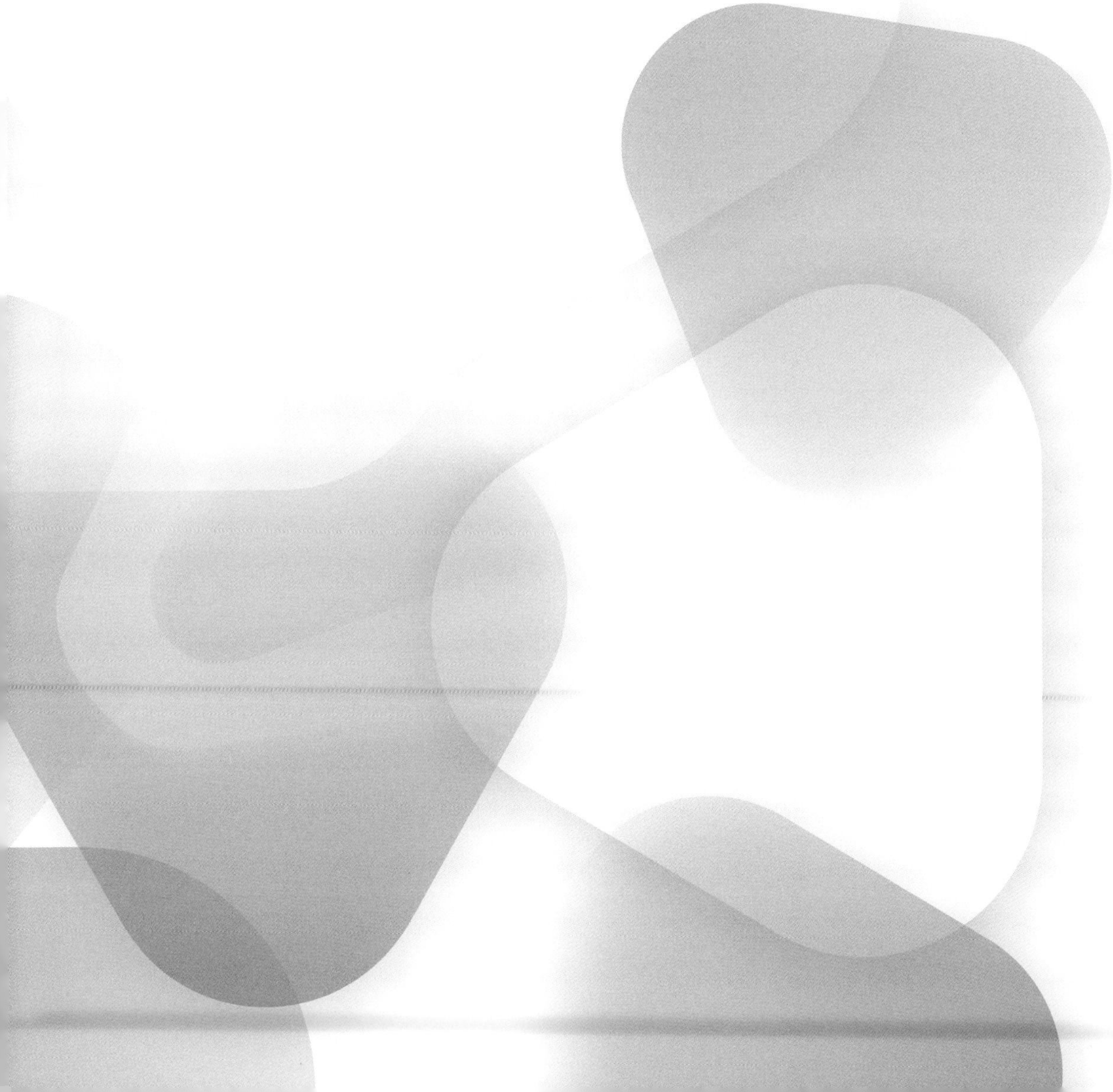

11

THE TRY-IN APPOINTMENT

Within the context of the previously described clinical and laboratory procedures, the wax try-in appointment should not take much time at all. However, it is important to thoroughly assess every aspect of the wax denture to avoid any laborious rework after implementation of the wax denture into acrylic. A diligent and precise workup makes the try-in appointment predictable.

The importance of having a close friend, family member, or life partner of the patient present at this appointment cannot be overstated.

Assessment of Function and Retention

It is recommended to check the functional aspects of the denture before moving to the esthetic evaluation. This avoids distractions greatly.

The previously disinfected wax dentures are once more rinsed under cold water. Because the setup was performed on the same record bases used during the last appointment, the fit and retention will only have improved due to the myofunctional wax-up, and surprises should not be expected here.

The maxillary wax denture is inserted first, and retention is tested by pulling the denture down and forward in the area of the central incisors. Next, the mandibular denture is inserted.

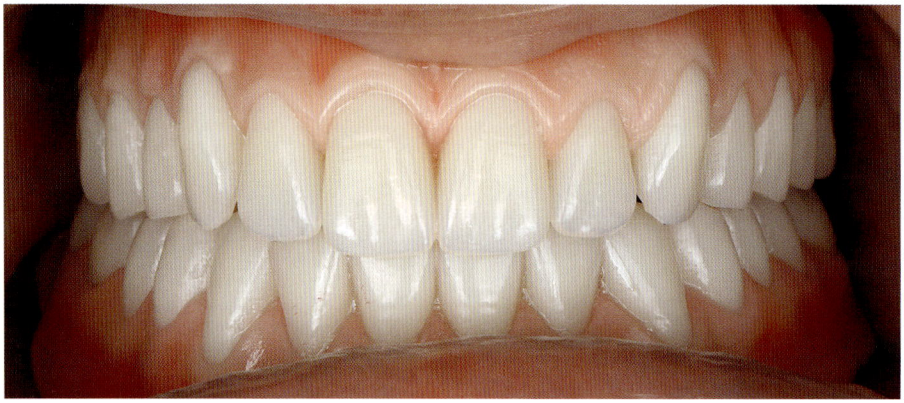

FIG 11-1 Occlusal function is assessed first visually, then with articulating silk.

The patient is asked to gently close into maximal intercuspation (MIP) and relax their lips. The vertical dimension and lip and cheek support are assessed. If satisfactory, the patient is asked to drink a small sip of water from a cup and remain in MIP. The clinician will then inspect the intercuspation, first visually and then by using occlusion foil or silk, ideally not thicker than 80 microns (Fig 11-1). Accurate records, mounting, and setting will result in evenly marked tripodized occlusal contacts between every antagonistic pair of posterior teeth.

Once the static contacts are confirmed, the clinician will insert a cotton roll, guide it between each pair of antagonistic teeth, and ask the patient to bite onto it (Fig 11-2). This will simulate actual unilateral mastication, and the clinician can observe any potential movement of either denture on the contralateral side. Any rotations, thrusts, or dislodgements need to be noted and evaluated. The cause must be identified clearly and communicated to the dental technician for remediation.

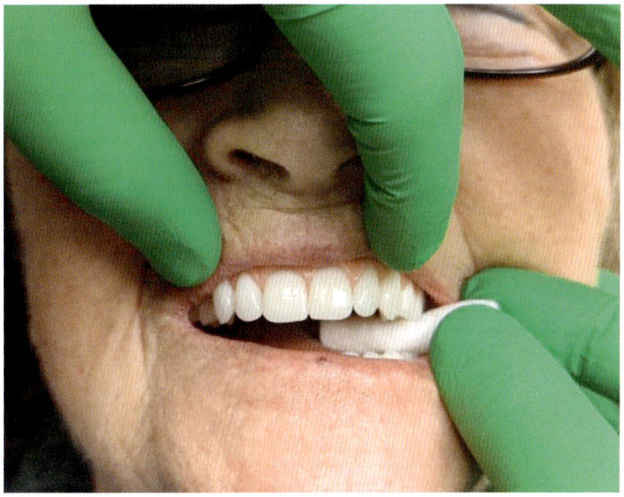

FIG 11-2 Positional stability is best tested with the patient biting on a cotton roll between each pair of antagonistic teeth.

Assessment of Phonetics

After the evaluation of function and positional stability, the phonetics must be evaluated. If any problems are detected, the cause must be identified.

A series of more targeted phonetic exercises may be used. The following words and phrases cover a wide area of phonetics and should be used for the formal evaluation:

- "M, M, church"
- Counting quickly from 1 to 10
- "Vivian" and "Vanessa"
- "Sheep" and "shepherd"
- "55, 66, 77"
- "Mississippi"
- "Then" and "there"
- "Monday, Monday, Monday"

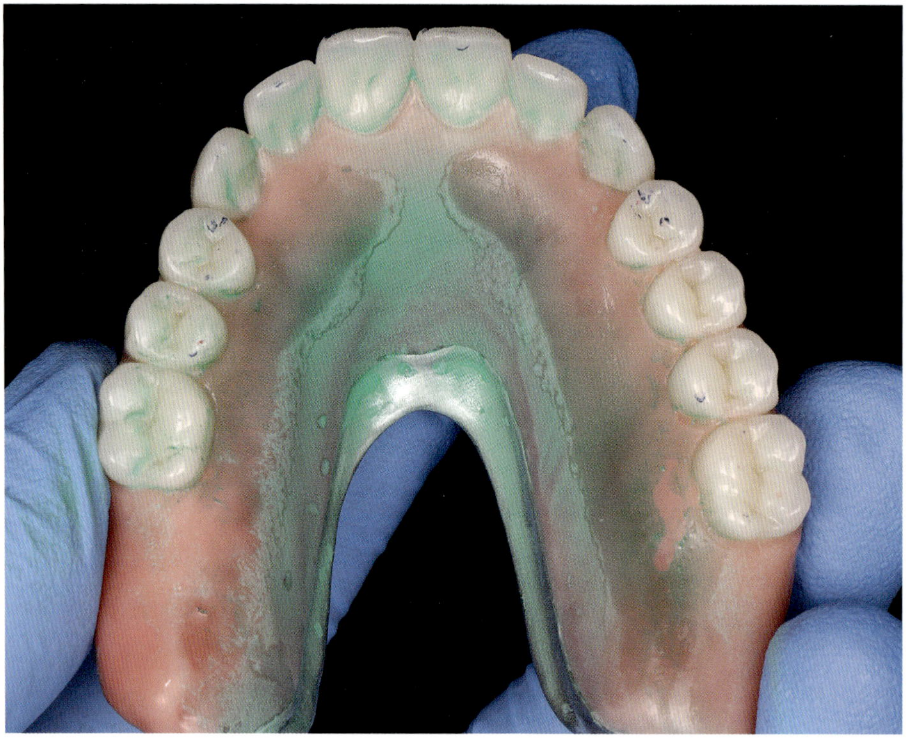

FIG 11-3 A palatogram can reveal the source of phonetic issues.

The clinician may apply contact spray to the palate of the wax trial to create a palatogram in order to identify problem areas (Fig 11-3). Small discrepancies may be remedied by adding or removing wax chairside. Here, close communication with the laboratory technician is of the utmost importance.

If the formal phonetic evaluation is satisfactory, the clinician will start a casual conversation with the patient. Ideally, this conversation is recorded with a video. This measure serves two purposes: *(1)* It can serve as a troubleshooting tool in case of difficulties with pronunciation. *(2)* It can be given to the patient to evaluate the prosthesis under relaxed conditions at home and can also be shared with loved ones before the wax dentures are resubmitted to the laboratory for processing.

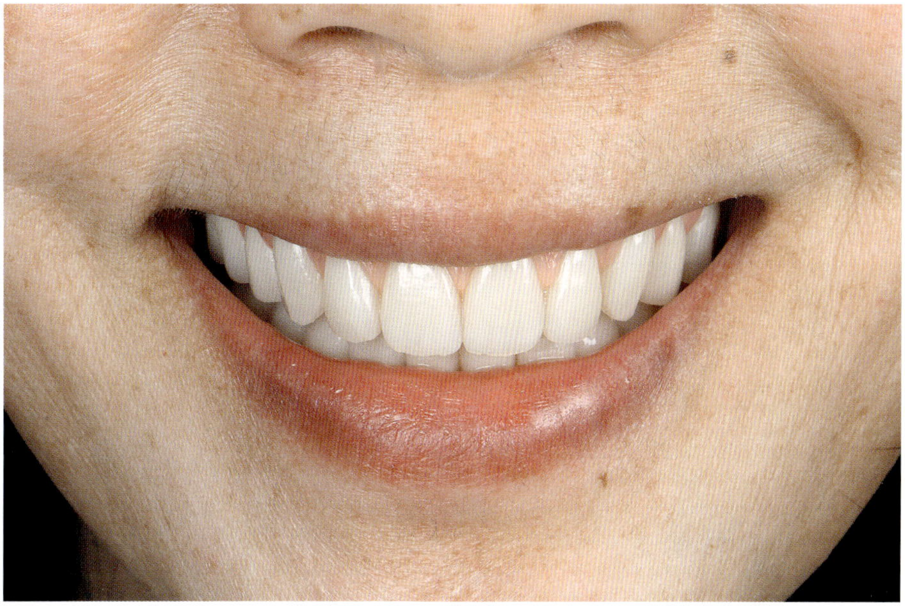

FIG 11-4 The final esthetic evaluation.

Assessment of Esthetics

Deliberately left as the final step of the try-in appointment, the patient is given time to evaluate their new smile (Fig 11-4). For this purpose, the patient is asked to step up to a wall-mounted large mirror to smile and talk. A smaller, handheld mirror can cause the patient to become distracted with insignificant details and prevent them from assessing their entire dentofacial appearance.

It can be valuable for the clinician to leave the operatory for a few minutes so that the patient and dental assistant can discuss the esthetics.

A written checklist or form for this appointment has proven valuable. It allows the clinical team to track every step of the appointment and note any potential changes for the dental laboratory technician (Fig 11-5).

Please use the following table to efficiently evaluate your denture try-in.

	No change	Needs change
Vertical dimension		
Lip support/phonetics		
Incisal edge position		
Midline		
Smile composition		
Size and shape of teeth		
Anterior and posterior occlusal plane		
Tooth shade		

Photos enclosed:

☐ Full-face frontal (closed) ☐ Full-face frontal (smile) ☐ Profile smile

Setup or occlusal changes:

Additional notes:

FIG 11-5 Example form used to assess the denture try-in.

12

PROCESSING

Choice of Processing Method

There are several methods available for the implementation of the wax dentures into acrylic:

- Injecting (manually or automatic)
- Packing
- Pressing
- Pouring/casting

Expertly performed, most processing methods can result in a satisfactory product. The pouring method, however, should be viewed critically due to the inherent high amount of residual monomer and comparatively high rate of acrylic shrinkage.

The dental laboratory technician is encouraged to evaluate both the processing method and the material used based on a comparison of final material properties.

For many years, the author has used XPLEX acrylics pressed with the Polymaster flasking system (Candulor) for denture processing, and the steps are described below. This material is a dual-curing high-impact PMMA with excellent flexural strength and colorfastness.

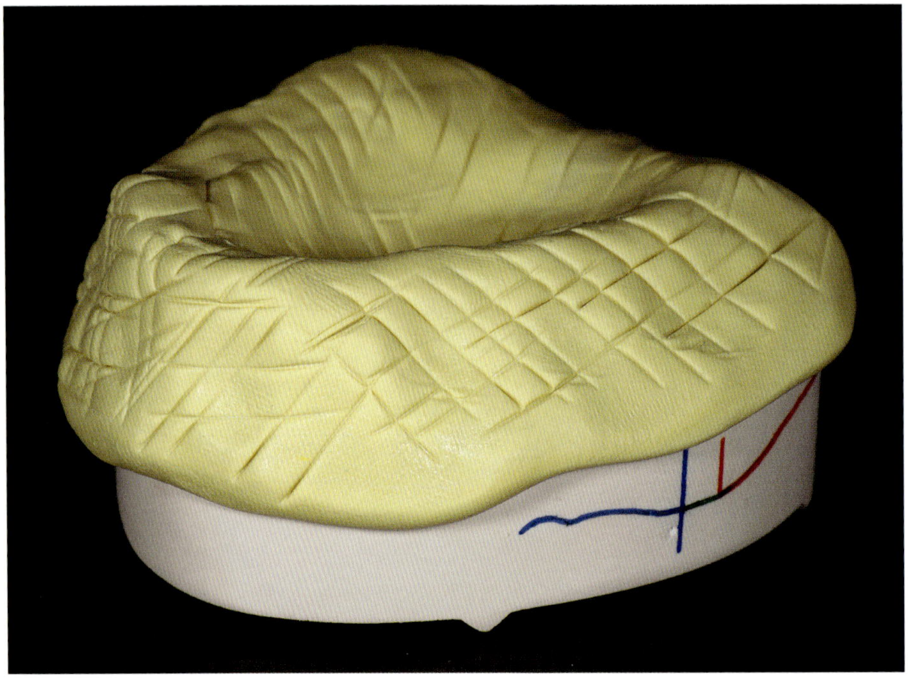

FIG 12-1 Primary silicone matrix to preserve the fine details of the wax-up and to protect the teeth during processing.

Investing with the Polymaster Flask

Once returned from the clinic, the wax dentures are diligently inspected for any potential damage. The occlusion is once more checked in the articulator before the record bases are sealed neatly onto the master cast. **Attention to detail during the model fabrication steps now pays dividends.**

An addition-type silicone putty with a higher shore hardness, like Sil-Tek Super (Ivoclar) is used to create a primary matrix, covering the teeth and wax-up. Once set, the matrix is carefully removed and a wash of light-bodied addition-type silicone, such as Flexistone Plus (DETAX), is applied before the primary matrix is seated on the wax denture once more. This method initially seems time- and cost-intensive but protects the denture teeth during processing and makes subsequent finishing extremely efficient (Figs 12-1 and 12-2).

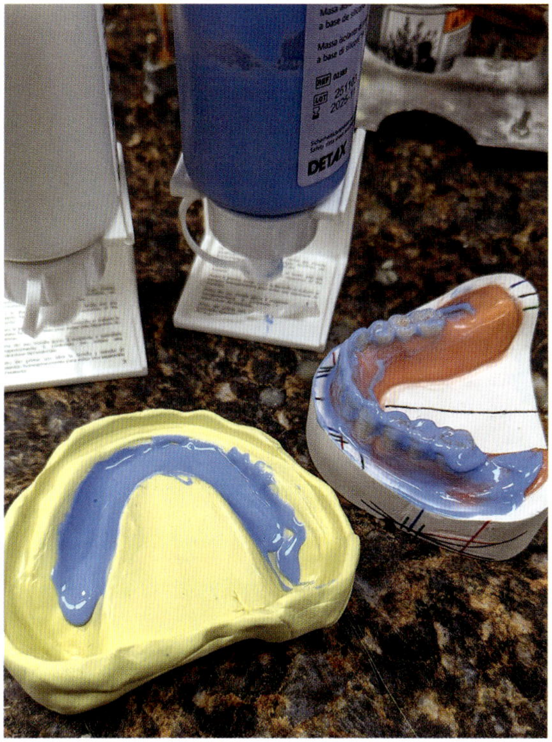

FIG 12-2 A flowable A-type silicone preserves the finest details of the wax model.

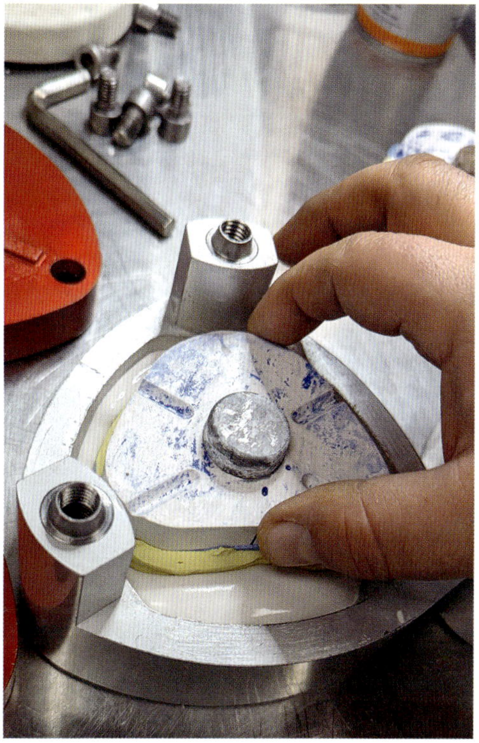

FIG 12-3 Investment in the Polymaster flask with an ISO Type 4 gypsum stone.

After the two-step matrix has completely set and any excess has been trimmed with a sharp knife, the models are invested in the Polymaster flask with an ISO Type 4 stone (Fig 12-3). The bottom surface of the model is then covered with a small amount of ISO Type 4 stone, and the top lid of the Polymaster flask is closed. Depending on experience, both the investment and counterinvestment may be completed in one step, or they can be completed separately. The stone investment must be allowed to fully set before the boil-out procedure begins.

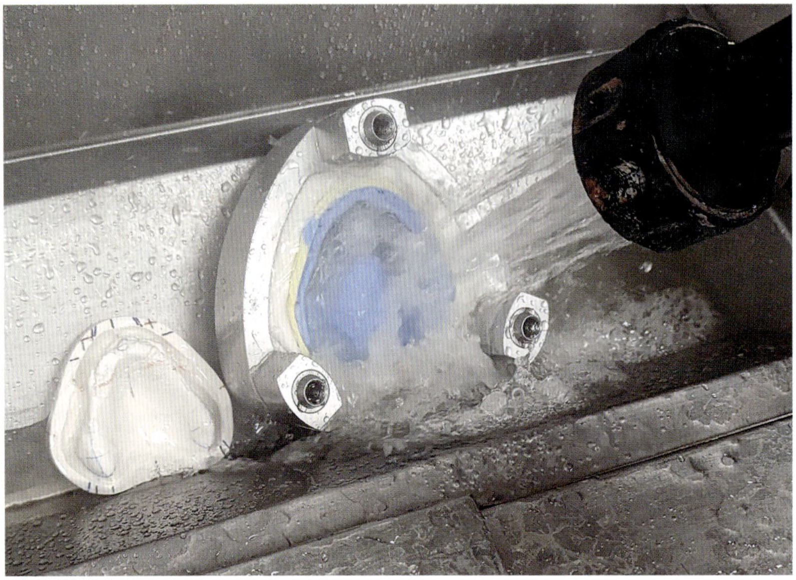

FIG 12-4 After the pre–boil-out, the opened flask and model is rinsed with hot water to remove any traces of residual wax.

Boil-out Procedure

A common mistake during the processing of acrylic is overheating of the flask, for example by placing the closed flask into a boil-out machine. If the wax is allowed to liquify, the stone surface will absorb it due to a wicking effect. The contaminated stone surface can hardly be cleaned again; even steam cleaning will only drive the wax particles deeper into the surface of the stone. The result is an unreliable insulation at subsequent steps.

It is therefore advisable to submerge the closed flask into a warm water bath or polymerization unit at 50°C for no more than 15 minutes. This method will plasticize the wax for clean and easy removal without allowing it to contaminate the stone surface.

After the pre–boil-out, the flask is opened and any larger portions of wax along with the record base are removed and discarded. A gentle stream of hot water will rinse any remaining wax from the investment and model (Fig 12-4).

Once cooled to a lukewarm temperature, an alginate-based isolation agent is applied in a thin layer to the stone surfaces with a clean, soft-bristled brush.

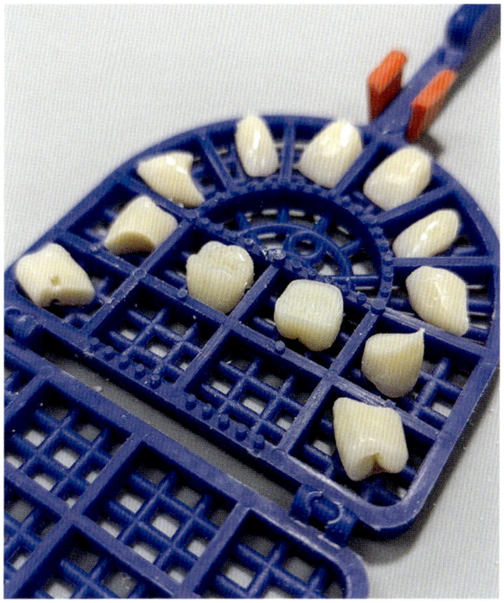

FIG 12-5 The teeth are removed from the silicone matrix and placed in a logical order into a tooth sieve, before the teeth are individually prepared for processing.

The first layer is allowed to air-dry for approximately 15 minutes, followed by a second very thin application. Any pooling of isolation fluid must be avoided. The second layer may be rinsed very briefly under a soft stream of water to achieve an exceptionally thin and smooth surface.

Preparation of the Denture Teeth

Ensuring a good chemical and mechanical bond between the denture teeth and the base acrylic is an important part of sensible craftsmanship. A diligent protocol here avoids delamination and warranty repairs, which are annoying for all involved. A proper bond also has hygienic advantages. Any experienced dental laboratory technician has seen dentures with discolorations and accumulations of biomaterials in the areas where the teeth and the base acrylic join.

The creation of vertical retention holes in the denture teeth is nonsense, as it inevitably creates air pockets and does virtually nothing in terms of mechanical retention, actually weakening the integrity of the denture tooth.

Rather, the teeth are removed from the silicone matrix and placed in a logical order into a tooth sieve (Fig 12-5). Tooth by tooth, the glaze on the

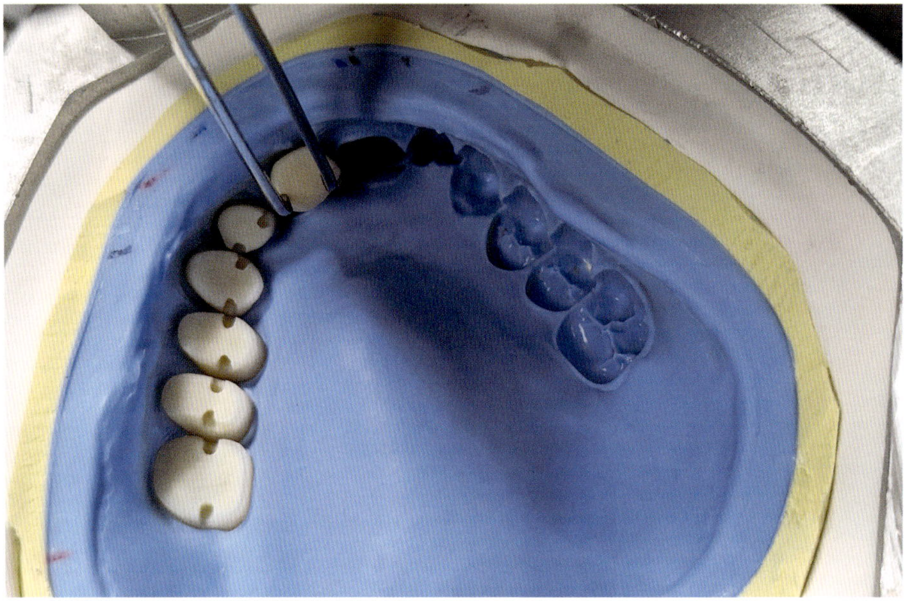

FIG 12-6 The teeth are returned to the matrix after deglazing and the application of mechanical retention grooves.

base of the teeth is removed with a crosscut carbide bur. Then a small notch is cut following the direction of the central fossa on the basal side (Fig 12-6). A reverse cone–shaped carbide bur works well here. Once each tooth has been prepared as described, the base of the tooth—including the cervical portion of the tooth later in contact with base acrylic—is treated with a sandblaster and 110-micron aluminum oxide. Finally, the teeth are cleaned with a steam cleaner. Care must be taken to avoid touching the teeth at this point without gloves, as the oils naturally occurring on the skin can contaminate the tooth and create a barrier, preventing a good chemical bond.

The teeth are placed securely back into the silicone matrix. Within 3 minutes before introducing the base acrylic, the teeth are wetted with the appropriate monomer for priming.

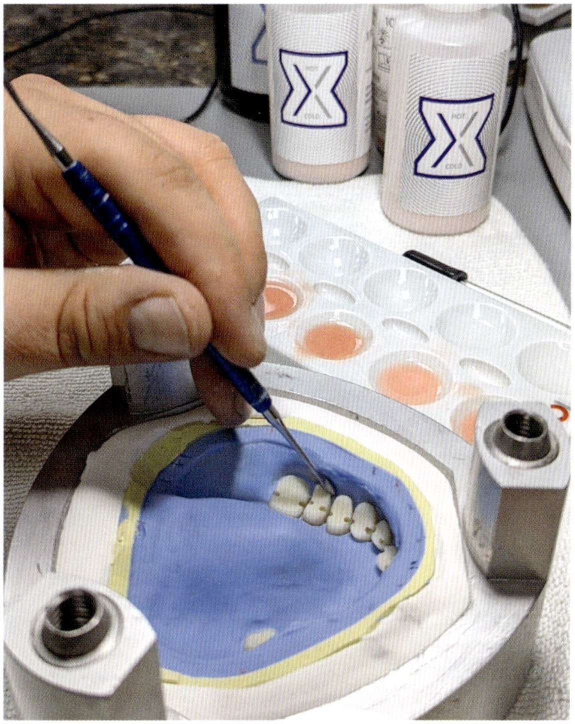

FIG 12-7 Gingival coloration within the flask.

Coloration of the Denture Base

As discussed in previous chapters, a polychromatic design of the denture base is an important part of a lifelike prosthesis. A uniform, artificial-looking pink shade of the gingiva will hardly create a natural appearance. While a cutback method and subsequent application of different colors of acrylic or composite are becoming more popular, the intrinsic staining of the denture base with specifically developed pigmented polymers has several advantages. Not only is this approach efficient and timesaving, but the application in the flask and use of a chemically identical material makes the effect colorfast, long-lasting, and hygienic (Fig 12-7).

The method requires some practice to achieve a well-blended, natural-looking end result, but this is well worth the effort. Preshaded kits are available, like the Aesthetic Color Set Easy (Candulor).

The base material is to be prepared and measured beforehand.

Pressing with XPLEX Autopolymerizing PMMA

Immediately after the intrinsic colorations are applied, the measured base material is mixed with a spatula for 30 seconds and allowed to mature for about 15 seconds. The total working time lasts approximately 1.5 to 3 minutes but can vary based on ambient temperature. Within this window of time, the material is filled into the flask and the lower lying areas of the model. Once the material has matured, the bottom plate of the Polymaster with the model is repositioned. The three Allen screws of the flasking system allow for gradual tightening and closing. It is recommended to tighten the screw facing the lip shield first. This prevents a potential displacement of the previously applied colors. After a transition phase of approximately 4 minutes, the flask must be fully closed.

Polymerization takes place in a polymerization unit for 15 minutes at a temperature of 50°C/122°F and under constant pressure of 2–6 bar/29–87 psi.

Deflasking

Regardless of the processing method used, the flask must always be allowed to bench cool to room temperature before deflasking. Immersion into cold water to speed up the process is not recommended, as this may lead to microfractures.

After cooling, the Allen screws are removed and the counterinvestment is freed from the top part of the flask with a plastic mallet. The remaining investment stone is removed with an air-chisel or nippers. The model is to remain intact, and its base is cleaned with a steam cleaner or a soft brush under running water.

13

FINISHING

Remount and Equilibration

Thanks to the secondary, magnetic split cast of the master models (see chapter 3), the remount into the articulator is seamless (Fig 13-1). The next step is the evaluation and equilibration of all static and dynamic occlusal contacts. While all dynamic or excursive contacts have been considered during the setup of the teeth in wax, the true creation of individual polyvalent occlusal geometry begins here. This process is also referred to as *selective grinding*. The protocol described below refers to the Condyloform II NFC+ posterior teeth.

It is important to understand the differences between types of articulators. The author exclusively uses instruments with a double-conus joint design, like the CA 3.0 (Candulor) and the Gerber Condylator (Condylator). This particular design of the condylar joints allows for a more physiologic 3D Bennett movement (Fig 13-2), unlike other makes that feature a rod or ball construction.

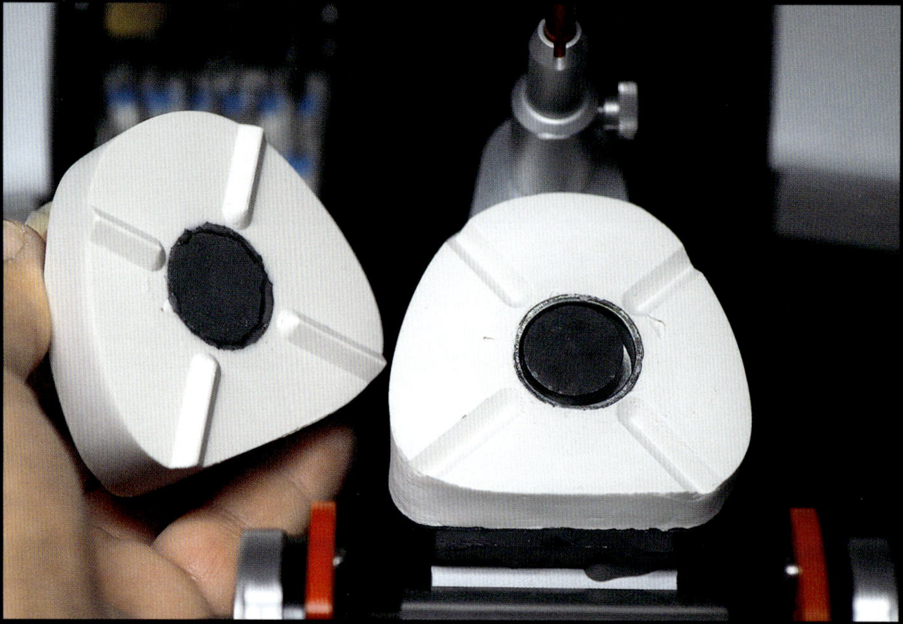

FIG 13-1 A magnetic split cast system makes setting the models back onto the mounting stone clean and precise.

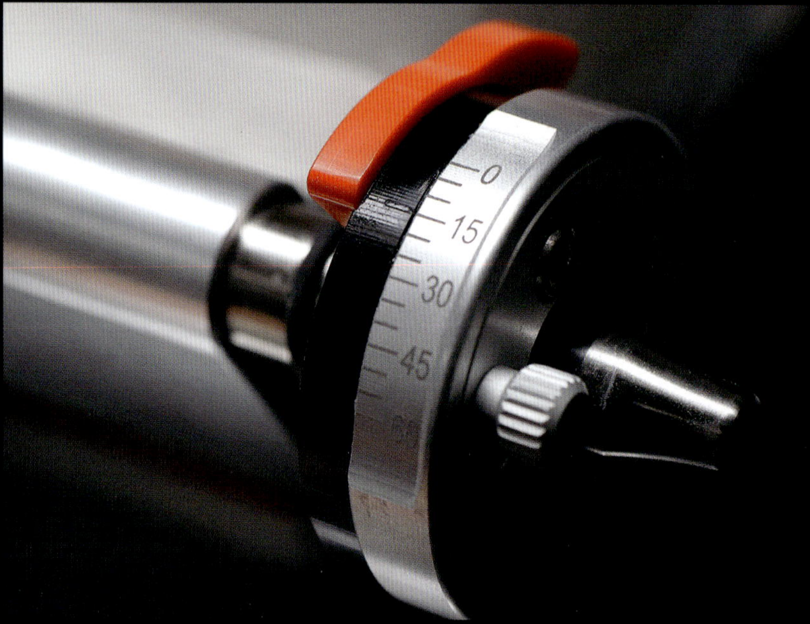

FIG 13-2 Articulators with a double-conus joint design allow for a more physiologic 3D Bennett movement.

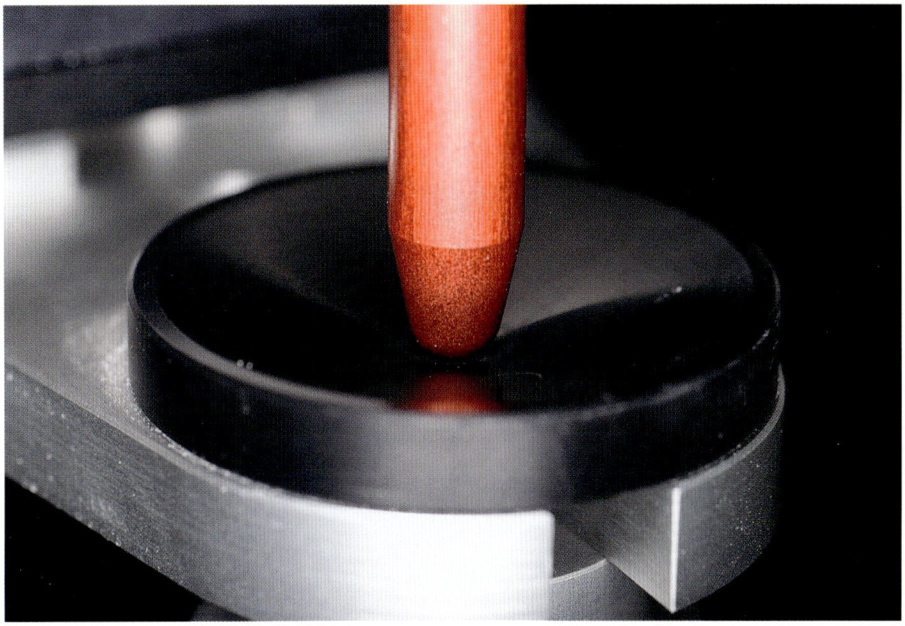

FIG 13-3 Dimensional changes that occur during processing can be identified by a raised pin.

Equilibration of Centric Contacts

With the condylar elements of the articulator in a locked position, the static occlusal contacts are checked with a red silk articulation ribbon. The incisal pin should have contact with the incisal guide plate. Dimensional changes that occur during processing can be identified by a raised pin. This is typically evident by hyperocclusions in the terminal posterior teeth.

Any vertical changes of more than 0.5-mm opening of the incisal pin, or any non-occlusion on specific teeth, should be considered a result of processing errors (Fig 13-3). In this case, resetting of the affected teeth may be indicated.

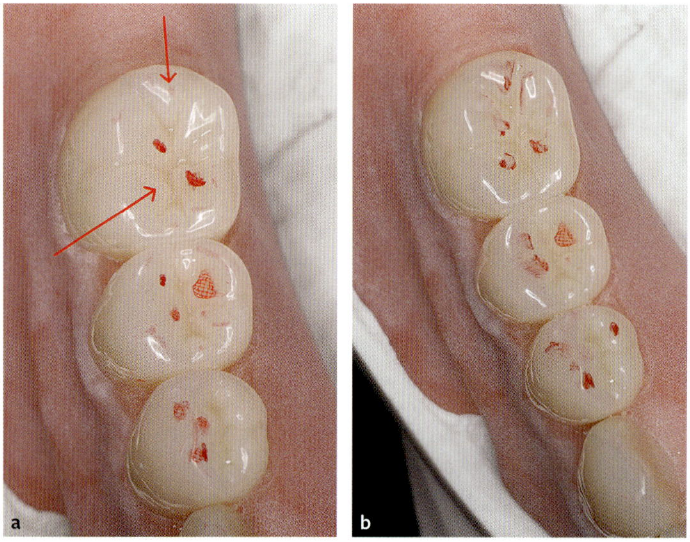

FIG 13-4 (*a*) Missing centric contacts (*arrows*). (*b*) Correct centric contacts on the mandibular posterior teeth are now visible after a minor adjustment.

Very small discrepancies are remedied with a small, round carbide or diamond bur (Fig 13-4). However, the following areas are NOT TO BE ground on:

- **Maxilla:**
  a. Palatal cusp of the first premolars
  b. Palatal cusp of the second premolars
  c. Mesiopalatal cusp of the first molars
  d. Mesiopalatal cusp of the second molars (if set up)
- **Mandible:** buccal cusp of the first premolars

The following areas MAY BE ground on:

- **Maxilla:** mesial central fossa of the first premolars
- **Mandible:**
  a. Distolingual fossa of the first premolars
  b. Central fossa of the second premolars
  c. Central fossa of the first molars
  d. Central fossa of the second molars (if set up)

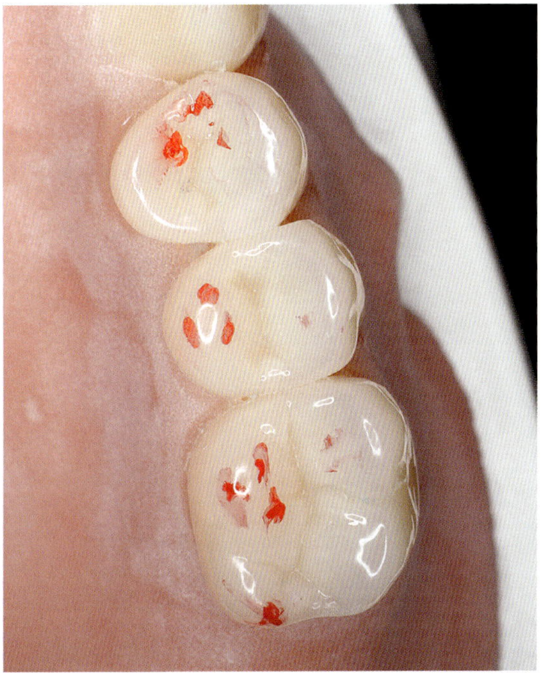

FIG 13-5 Correct centric contacts on the maxillary posterior teeth.

The goal is to achieve three points of centric contact (tripodization) on each posterior tooth (Fig 13-5). This is the prerequisite for bilaterally balanced occlusion, which is described in the next steps. It can be advantageous to mark the final centric contacts with a red fine-point permanent marker.

Equilibration of the Protrusion

The condylar elements are programmed to their individual values. These values have been obtained with a protrusive record, or via condylography, as described in chapter 4 (Figs 13-6 and 13-7). The condylar elements are unlocked on both sides, and a green silk articulation ribbon is used to mark a protrusive movement of approximately 3 mm. The goal is to create protrusive tracks on each posterior tooth by selective grinding (Fig 13-8). To achieve this, the following areas MAY BE ground on:

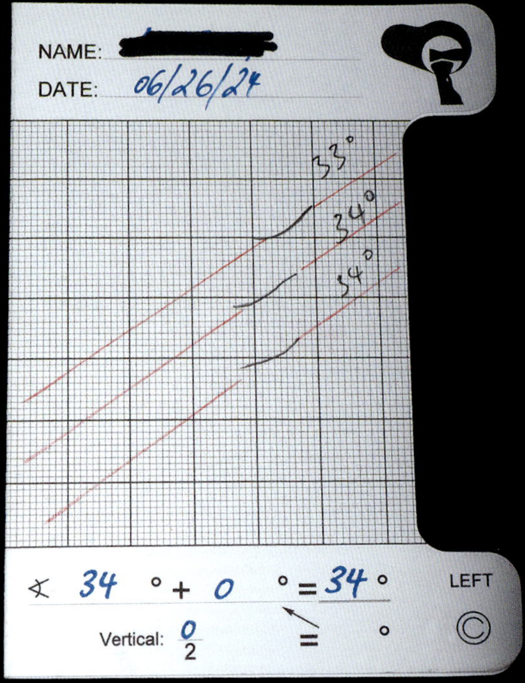

FIG 13-6 Evaluation of the condylography shows a sagittal condylar slope of 34 degrees.

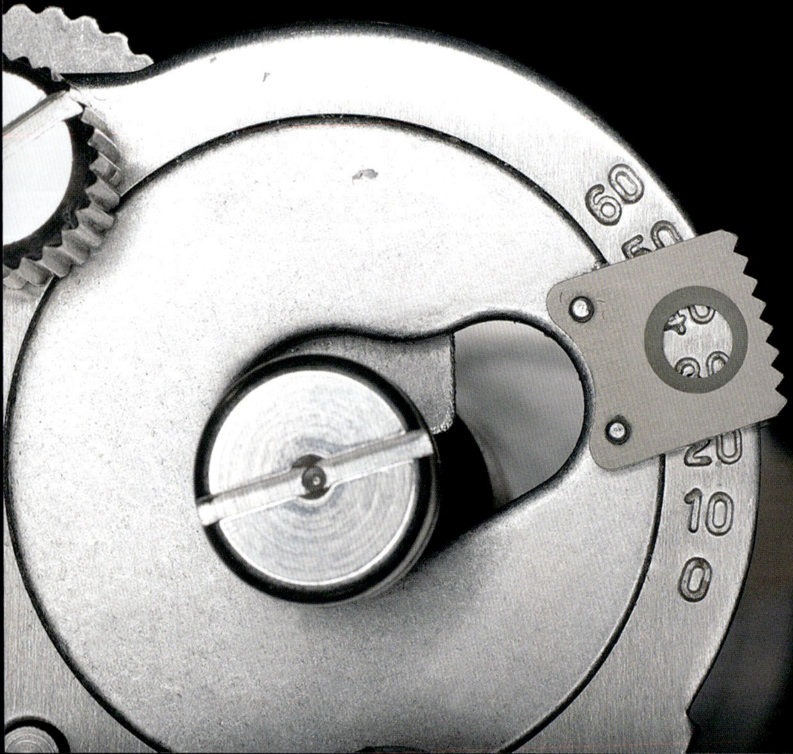

FIG 13-7 The condylar element of the Condylator is set to the correct value.

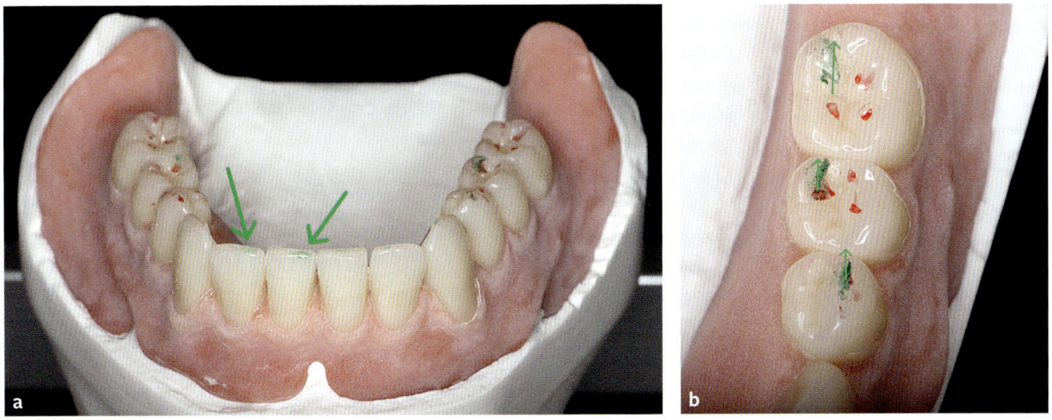

FIG 13-8 (*a*) Small guidances in the anterior region (*arrows*) prohibit full protrusive contacts on all posterior teeth. (*b*) All protrusive contacts (*arrows*) are now visible after selective reduction of the anterior guidances.

- **Maxilla:**
  a. Palatal surfaces of the incisors
  b. Distobuccal cusp of the first premolars
- **Mandible:**
  a. Labial surfaces of the incisors
  b. Distolingual of the first premolars to mesiolingual of the second premolars
  c. From the centric contact of the second premolars to the mesial ridge of the first molars
  d. From the centric contact of the first molars to distolingual
  e. From the centric contact of the second molars to distolingual

Equilibration of the Laterotrusion and Immediate Side Shift

The equilibration of the laterotrusion is always completed toward one side first. Once an interference-free movement is achieved, the process is repeated on the other side.

With the condylar element of the respective side unlocked, the laterotrusive movement is marked and equilibrated using a blue articulating ribbon. Once the procedure is completed, bilateral working and balancing contacts are clearly visible. The same principles apply as described above. Typically, hyper-guidances can be detected on the canines and maxillary first premolars. For a bilaterally balanced occlusion, these guidances must be eliminated, as canine and sequential guidance is typically not desired in conventional dentures.

The following areas MUST NOT be ground on:

- **Maxilla:**
  a. Palatal cusps of the first premolars
  b. Palatal cusps of the second premolars
  c. Palatal cusps of the first molars
  d. Palatal cusps of the second molars
- **Mandible:** buccal cusps of the first premolars

On the **working side**, the following areas MAY BE ground on (Fig 13-9):

- **Maxilla:** mesiobuccal cusps of the first premolars
- **Mandible:**
  a. From the centric contact of the second premolars to mesiolingual
  b. From the centric contact of the first molars to mesiolingual
  c. From the centric contact of the second molars to mesiolingual

On the **balancing side**, the following areas MAY BE ground on:

- **Maxilla:** from the centric contact of the first premolars to mesiobuccal
- **Mandible:**
  a. From the centric contact of the second premolars to distobuccal
  b. From the centric contact of the first molars to distobuccal
  c. From the centric contact of the second molars to distobuccal

Once the laterotrusive movements have been equilibrated bilaterally, both condylar elements are unlocked, and the immediate side shift is checked and equilibrated, if necessary, by shifting the articulator hinge sideways by 1.5 mm.

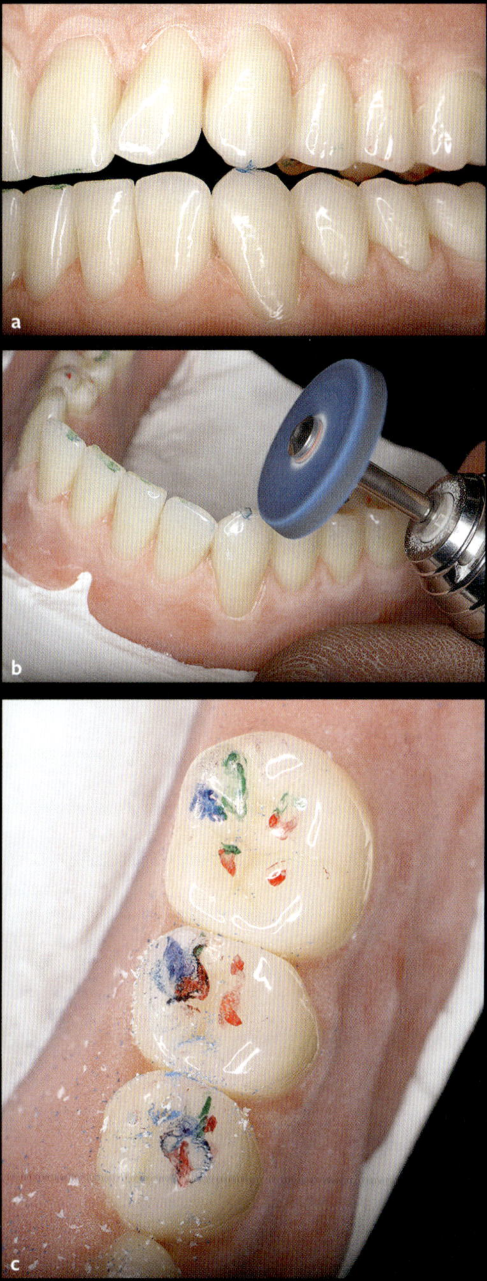

FIG 13-9 (*a*) Canine guidance prevents working-side contacts in laterotrusion to the left. (*b*) Removal of hyperguidance with a rubber wheel. (*c*) All working-side contacts in laterotrusion to the left are now visible.

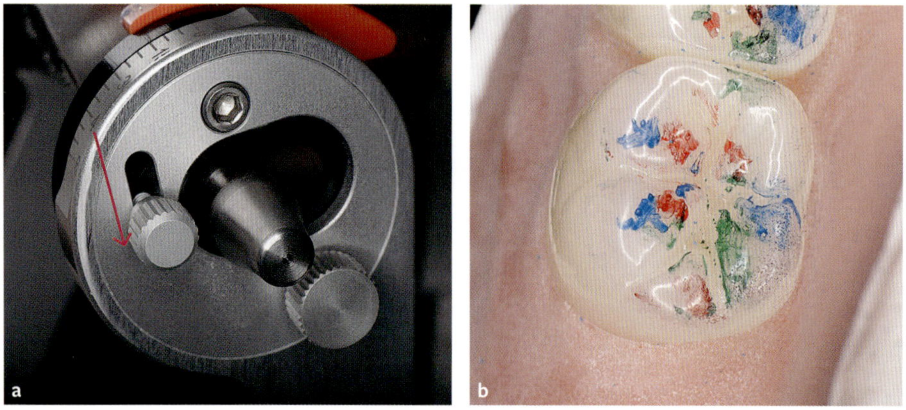

FIG 13-10 (*a*) Retrusion lock on the CA 3.0 articulator in the unlocked position (*arrow*). (*b*) Functionally complete equilibration of a mandibular left first molar.

Equilibration of the Retrusion

Many common articulators are not capable of simulating a retrusive movement, or they do so in a nonphysiologic fashion. The retrusive range of the temporomandibular joint from physiologic centric relation is typically extremely short (1.0–1.5 mm) and describes a dorsal/caudal path. If the instrument used allows for a physiologic reproduction of the retrusive movement, equilibration is recommended to eliminate potential gliding obstacles mesial to the centric contacts in the mandible (Fig 13-10).

Finishing and Polishing

Once the equilibration is completed, the dentures are freed from the models with an air-chisel or nippers. Care must be taken to avoid creating torsion, which could fracture the base acrylic.

With a highly detailed wax-up and a diligent processing procedure, finalizing the prosthesis is fast and efficient (Fig 13-11). Fine-cut carbide burs of multiple shapes and sizes as well as sandpaper strips are recommended. Rubber polishers tend to produce too much heat and can deform the acrylic. A 5-mm-diameter, double-sided diamond disc is used to remove thin acrylic flash between the teeth.

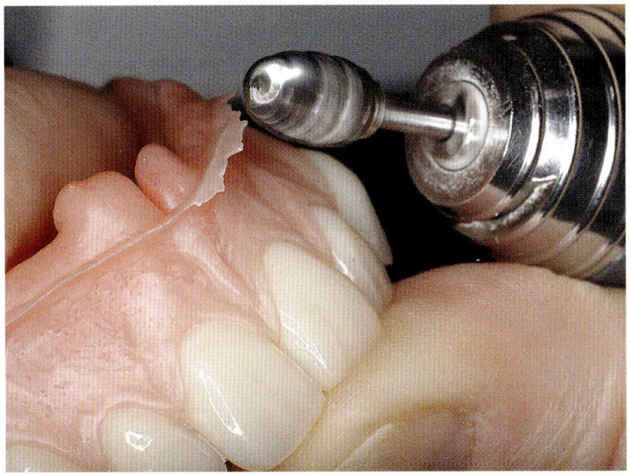

FIG 13-11 A detailed wax-up and clean processing now pays dividends. The small press vane (flash) is blended into the denture body.

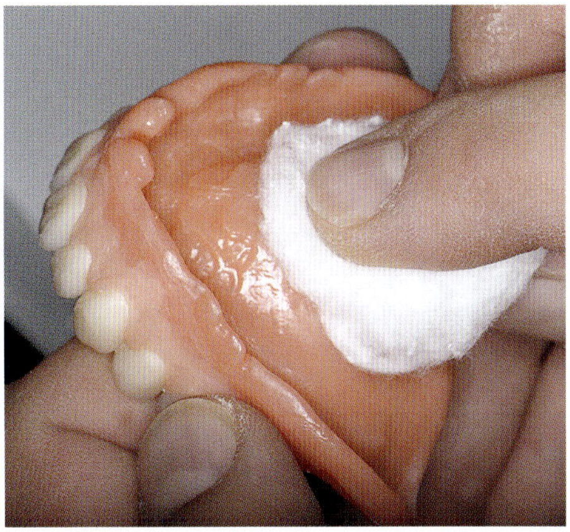

FIG 13-12 A cotton ball is used to detect even the smallest beads or sharp areas on the intaglio surface.

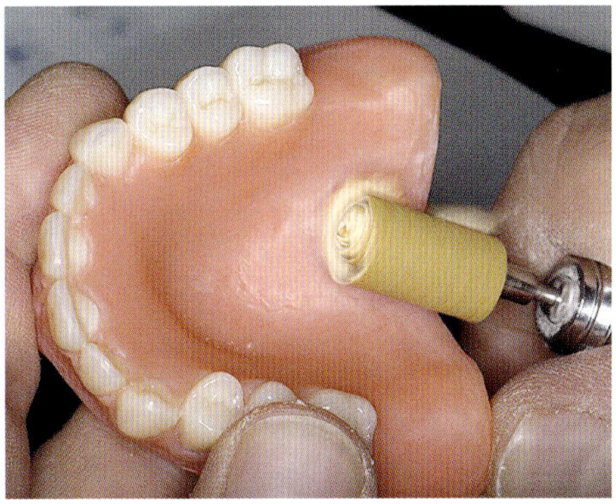

FIG 13-13 Rotating sandpaper strips mounted on special mandrels are used to gently blend any sharp or uneven areas.

Any beads caused by small bubbles in the model or sharp edges on the intaglio surface are detected using a cotton ball (Fig 13-12). These are then carefully removed with a small bur. Next, the press vane formed along the model margins is carefully removed without changing the shape of the outer valve margin. Rotating sandpaper strips mounted on special mandrels are used to gently blend any sharp or uneven areas (Fig 13-13). The dorsal border of the maxillary denture is gently tapered to a point.

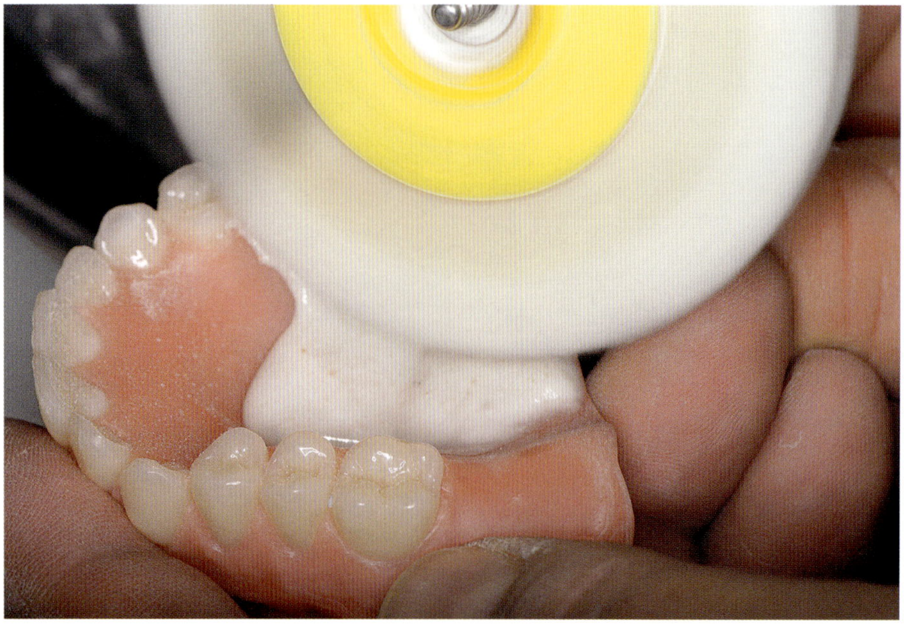

FIG 13-14 Larger areas may be polished at the lathe with pumice or pumice substitute and a larger brush wheel on low speed.

The valve margins were already established during the functional impressions, and to ensure a good seal, **they must not be altered!** This includes the passages of the frenulae. A random alteration of these areas can ruin the suction effectiveness of the dentures and must be strictly avoided.

A caliper should be used to check the minimum thickness of the denture base. There should be no areas thinner than 1.75 mm.

Larger areas, such as the palate and the lingual denture body, may be polished with pumice or pumice substitute and a Chungking brush wheel mounted on a lathe (Fig 13-14).

All other areas, including the functional borders, should be polished with a goat-hair brush wheel and polishing compound on the handpiece (Figs 13-15 and 13-16). Pumice and rag wheels are too abrasive and can significantly alter the valve margins and destroy fine anatomical details on teeth and the lip shield. A small chamois cloth or soft leather buff is used for the high shine (Fig 13-17), followed by a final pass with a small cotton buff (Fig 13-18).

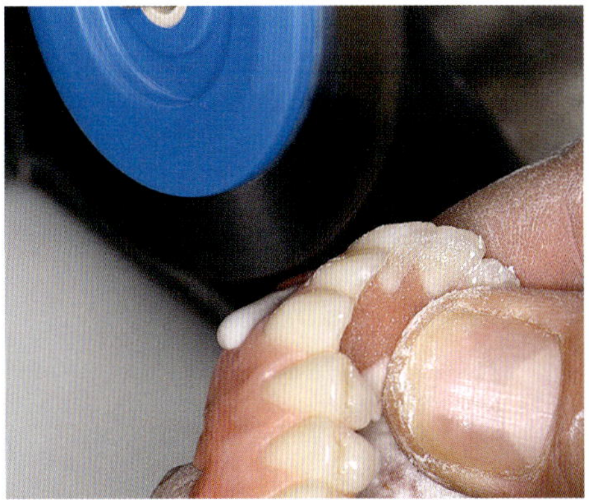

FIG 13-15 Smaller areas are polished with pumice or pumice substitute and a small soft brush.

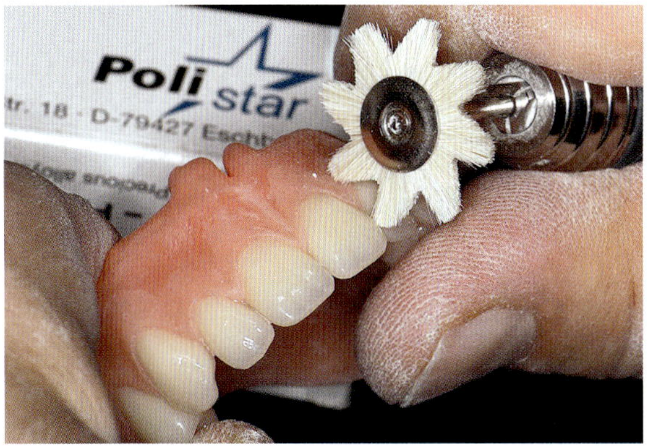

FIG 13-16 A small goat-hair bush wheel is used at 5,000 revolutions per minute (rpm) with polishing compound to polish the smallest details and the valve margins.

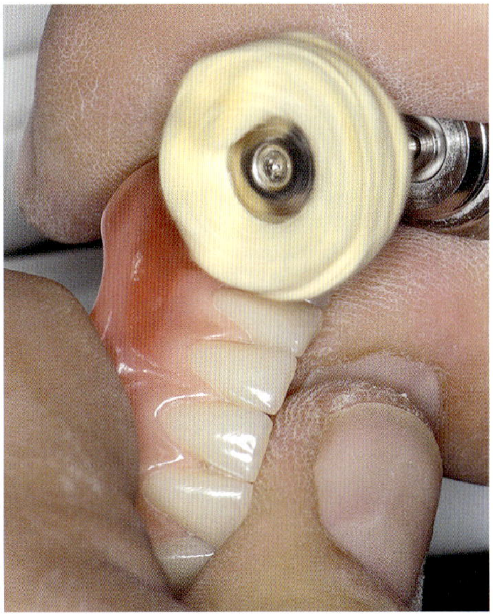

FIG 13-17 A leather buff at 5,000 rpm with a small amount of KMG Paste (Candulor) is used on and around the teeth.

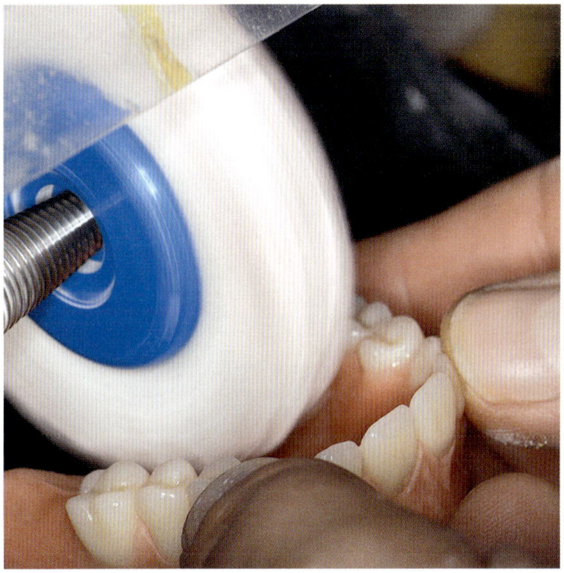

FIG 13-18 The final high shine is achieved with a very soft cotton wheel at low speed on the lathe with a small amount of high-shine KMG Liquid (Candulor).

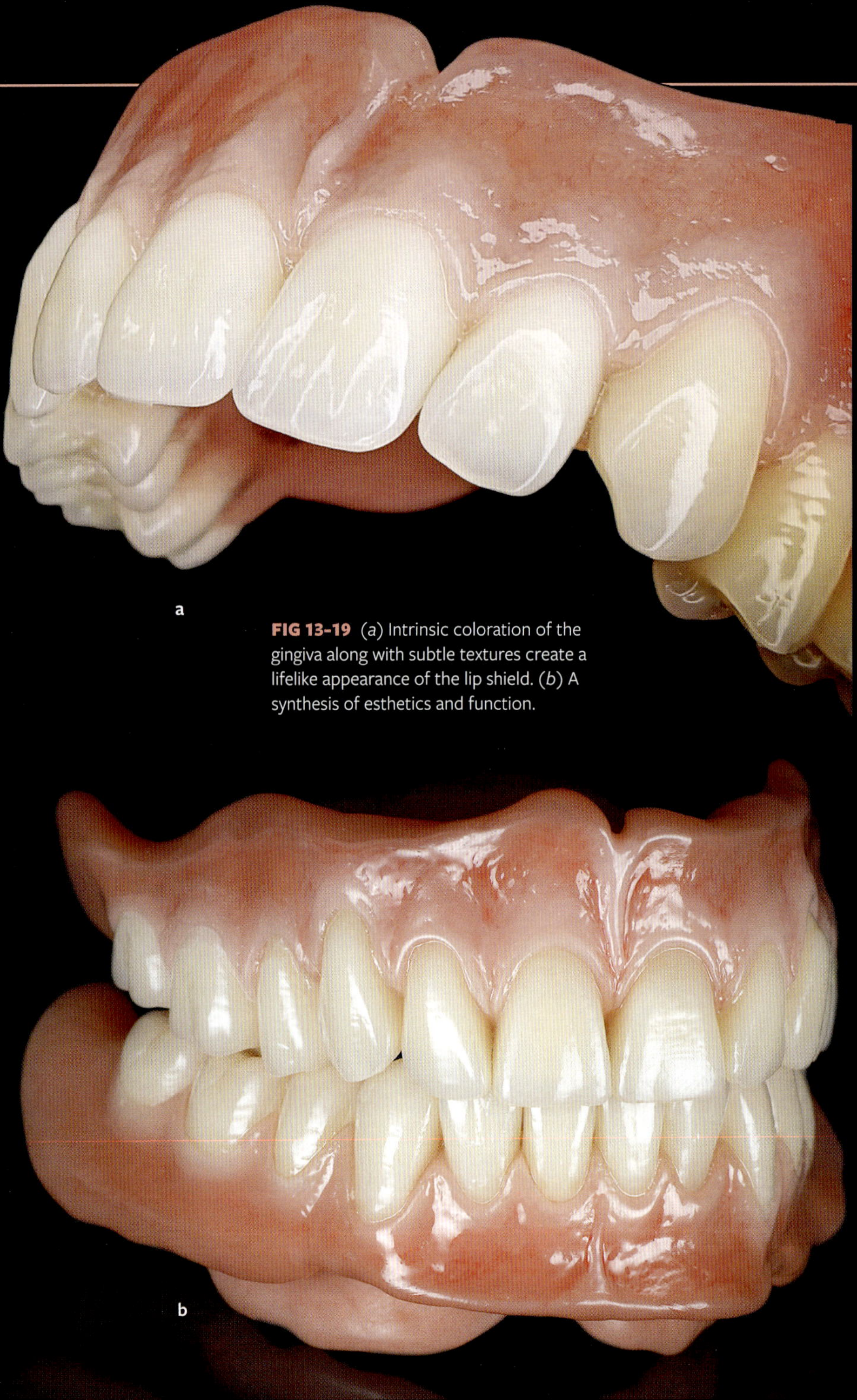

a

FIG 13-19 (*a*) Intrinsic coloration of the gingiva along with subtle textures create a lifelike appearance of the lip shield. (*b*) A synthesis of esthetics and function.

b

A thorough cleaning of the final dentures in an ultrasonic unit is followed by a final quality-control protocol (Fig 13-19).

CLOSING WORDS

Prosthetics and the Human Being

As mentioned in the beginning of this book, a *prosthetic* is, by definition, an artificial body part, such as a leg, a heart, or a denture. As is the case with all other types of prosthetics, dentures require time to allow the body to accept the artificial part, and a symbiosis can only be achieved if the patient is willing to consistently practice with it. It would be unrealistic to expect to comfortably eat a T-bone steak the day of delivery.

Here, the clinician must play a pivotal role: The goals and challenges of the treatment plan must be clearly understood by the patient even before the primary impressions are taken. This requires empathy and sensitivity. The patient is not only the center of all efforts by the treatment team but also a part of it. Even the most sophisticated prosthetics do not work without the patient's cooperation and willingness to adapt.

Prosthetics and Digital Technology

Newly evolving digital workflows are becoming more common in dental treatment. To fully reject these advancements in technology is as absurd as the uncritical adaptation of new technologies for their own sake.

The treatment team must evaluate new tools—digital or otherwise—and their usefulness in achieving prosthetic success sensibly. The principles described in the preceding pages are based on scientific facts and decades of experience. Human physiology, anatomy, and ultimately psychology have not changed. As long as a new technology can accommodate or improve a workflow, it should be viewed with curiosity—but always from an educated perspective and with the patient in mind. **The patient should be at the heart of everything we do.**

BIBLIOGRAPHY

Abe J, Iwaki K, Sudo T, Kokubo K. Mandibular Suction-Effective Denture: "The Professional." Quintessence, 2017.

Berry FH. Is the theory of temperament the foundation to the study of prosthetic art? Dent Mag 1905;1:405.

Bosshart M. Funktion and Ästhetik: Rehabilitation des Unbezahnten nach der Original-Gerber-Methode. Quintessence, 2014.

Frush JP. A study of the dentogenetic concept of dental esthetics and dynesthetics. Swissedent Foundation, 1957.

Frush JP, Fisher RD. Introduction to dentogenetic restorations. J Prosthet Dent 1955;5:586–595.

Gerber A. Basic aesthetics in complete dentures. Quintessence Int 1975.

Gerber A. Beiträge zur totalen Prothese (I–VIII). Teil VI: Prinzipielles zur Bißnahme für totale Prothesen. Die Quintessenz 1973;8:599–601.

Gerber A. Proportionen und Stellung der Frontzähne im natürlichen und künstlichen Zahnbogen. Die Quintessenz 1965;16:33–42.

Gerber A. Statik, Artikulation und Gestaltung des Kauflaechenkomplexes. Schweiz Monatssch Zahnheilk 1955.

Gerber A, Preti G. Kaudynamik—Funktionen, die funktionieren muessen [video]. Quintessence, 2006.

Gerber A, Steinhardt G. Dental Occlusion and the Temporomandibular Joint. Quintessence, 1990.

Gysi A. Das Aufstellen einer ganzen Prothese. Schweiz Vrtjhrschr Zahnheilk 1915.

Kimoto S, Gunji A, Yamakawa A, et al. Prospective clinical trial comparing lingualized occlusion to bilateral balanced occlusion in complete dentures: A pilot study. Int J Prosthodont 2006;19:103–109.

Lerch P. Die totale Prothetik. Quintessence, 1986.

Shafie HR. Clinical and Laboratory Manual of Implant Overdentures. Wiley, 2013.

Stuck J, Horn R. Zahnaufstellung in der Totalprothetik. Quintessence, 1980.

Sülün T, Ergin U, Tuncer N. The nose shape as a predictor of maxillary central and lateral width. Quintessence Int 2005;36:603–607.

INDEX

Page references followed by "f" denote figures.